41210 (1)

THE SPINE AND
MEDICAL NEGLIGENCE

R.W. Porter

Formerly Professor of Orthopaedic Surgery,
University of Aberdeen, UK
and
Director of Education and Training,
The Royal College of Surgeons, Edinburgh, UK

βIOS
SCIENTIFIC
PUBLISHERS

Oxford • Washington DC

A CIP catalogue record for this book is available from the British Library.

ISBN 185996 126 6

BIOS Scientific Publishers Ltd
9 Newtec Place, Magdalen Road, Oxford OX4 1RE, UK
Tel. +44 (0)1865 726286 Fax +44 (0)1865 246823
World Wide Web home page: http://www.bios.co.uk

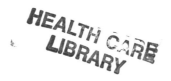

Production Editor: Andrea Bosher
Typeset by Marksbury Multimedia Ltd, Midsomer Norton, UK
Printed by Biddles Ltd, Guildford, UK

CONTENTS

SPINAL COMPLICATIONS

FOREWORD

It is a double pleasure to be asked to write this Foreword. In the first place, Professor Richard Porter is an outstanding clinician and teacher with the gift of clear exposition. Many will have heard him speak at the weekend conferences of the Professional Negligence Bar Association and Action for Victims of Medical Accidents. Secondly, he has an instinctive knowledge of what lawyers require in a medico-legal report. He has been of incomparable value in a number of cases in which I have been involved and we have an unbroken record of success. Now he produces a volume which comprehensively covers the medical and legal aspects of spinal surgery. Its contents will direct and educate both doctors and lawyers in a wide specialist area, where damages, if awarded, will often be substantial. The explanations, glossaries and references are especially valuable for both professions.

Richard Hone QC

ACKNOWLEDGEMENTS

I am indebted to my friend Richard Hone QC for writing a generous foreword. Three friends have supplied a number of illustrations in Chapters 5, 8 and 10 to 15. Dr Paul Butt is a consultant radiologist at St James University, Leeds and has allowed me to include many of his CT scans. Dr John A. McCulloch is Professor of Orthopaedic Surgery, Northeast Ohio Universities College of Medicine, USA and he has provided many excellent illustrations of MRI. Dr Francis W. Smith, MRI unit, Woodend Hospital, Aberdeen, UK has provided the bone scan images. I am grateful to them and to Churchill Livingstone for permission to include several illustrations previously used in my book *Management of Back Pain* (1993) 2nd edition, chapters 10, 11 and 12. I thank the Royal College of Surgeons of Edinburgh for photographs of two skeletons from their museum.

INTRODUCTION

The principal goal of every surgeon is to provide good quality care. Unfortunately there are occasions when they miss the mark, and a careful assessment of why things went wrong can then be helpful. Some patients believe that their treatment was below the standard expected, and they are justified. There are claims which have merit and others which seem frivolous. Most surgeons face claims of alleged negligence at some time during their career, and spinal surgeons are particularly vulnerable.

A strong wind of change is blowing through the practice of surgery. It affects surgeons and lawyers alike. A generation ago, doctors knew what was best for the patients, or they thought they did, and patients did as they were told. There were occasional mistakes but patients accepted that the doctor had always done his best. Allegations of medical negligence were uncommon. The sun shone in the sky, and surgeons could sleep in their beds.

Now, however, most doctors know the discomfort of being sued. There has been an exponential increase in litigation. The *Sunday Times* reported in November 1996 [1], under a heading 'Legal aid soars as Britons sue the American way', that the British legal aid bill had increased from £166m in 1990 to £544m in 1995. The government's bill for NHS indemnity had increased three-fold in those 5 years. The Medical Defence Union (MDU) reported a 50% increase in awards in the past 3 years, paying £67m in 1996 to defend accused doctors. Over £18m went in legal costs.

Many surgeons are learning not only new surgical skills, but also how to protect themselves from allegations of negligence and how to defend themselves in court. They have had to become alert to the dangers of transgression. They also recognize that there is a bonus. By understanding how these incidents occur, there is an opportunity to change practice and improve patient care. Surgeons and management alike have to take the observations of patients seriously. Claims of alleged negligence provide useful information about standards of care. If they result in an improvement in practice, this is more important than just conducting an exercise in customer relations.

From time to time mistakes will inevitably occur, but doctors hope that with goodwill and understanding on both sides – apologies and a genuine attempt to prevent a recurrence – this will satisfy the injured party, and it will not result in litigation. There are many patients who have the right to sue, and fail to do so. In the USA there are eight times as many acts of medical negligence as claims for compensation, and 14 claims for every successful claim [2, 3]. Thus, even in the litigious USA there is potential for more litigation than is currently experienced [4]. We need to understand why patients sue their doctor, but also why they do not sue when it would be justified. Most claims do not go to court. In one study only 11% of orthopaedic claims reached court and, of these, 85% resulted in a defence verdict; 56% of claims were withdrawn or dismissed and 31% were settled out of court [5].

The express provision of the legal aid scheme is that the litigation has to be justified. However, many doctors feel that there is an increasing number of unsubstantiated claims causing much wasted time. There is a view that British lawyers are now finding "ways of suing for almost any injury or slight however trivial" [1]. Doctors find themselves having to spend much time in the defence of unsuccessful claims, and in the development of undue protectionism. The time, cost and turmoil is often out of all proportion to any compensation due, or to the extent to which the public interest may be served by the outcome of any legal proceedings [6].

Spinal surgery is an important aspect of alleged negligence. In financial terms the defence of mismanaged spinal surgery is considerable. Spinal operations, when compared with other types of surgery, are associated with significantly high risk, and mismanaged spinal surgery is the most costly of all orthopaedic procedures to defend. The American Academy of Orthopaedic Surgeons reported that the average defence costs for an orthopaedic surgeon who performed spine surgery was US$49 837, whilst the defence costs of other orthopaedic procedures was half that amount [5].

In this book we shall be examining both general and specific issues of negligence. All medical specialities are interested in the general concepts of why patients sue their doctors, what is informed consent and reasonable risk management. These are important issues for all disciplines. We shall, however, also be addressing problems of negligence in relation to spine surgery. Allegations are frequently about lack of informed consent, technical complications and systems failure, poor surgical performance, misdiagnosis and failure to identify and manage a complication. In this book we shall be looking at these in detail.

There are a number of case studies which have been used to illustrate the complex problems of litigation. They all have an element of truth, but details have been changed to preserve anonymity. Some of the clinical information will be simplistic to the surgeon, but it has been included to help the lawyer who may not be so familiar with medical details. There is also a glossary of terms to help the non-medical reader. References are included for those who want to explore the medical literature in more detail.

Hopefully this book will assist surgeons and managers to reduce the risk of negligence claims. More importantly it might improve their clinical practice. The book is also written to help lawyers understand the particular problems and difficulties which face spinal surgeons, and when allegations of negligence are reasonable and when they are unjustified. We are exploring a difficult but important aspect of medico-legal practice.

REFERENCES

1. The *Sunday Times*, 17 November 1996.
2. Hiatt HH, Barnes BA, Brennan TA, *et al*. A study of medical injury and medical malpractice: an overview *New Eng. J. Med.* 1989; 321: 480.
3. Leape II, Brennan TA, Laird NM, *et al*. The nature of adverse events in hospitalized patients. *New Eng. J. Med.* 1991; 324: 377.
4. Vincent C, Young M, Phillips A. Why do people sue doctors? A study of patients and relatives taking legal action *The Lancet* 1994; 343: 1609–1613.
5. *Managing orthopaedic malpractice risk*. Prepared by the Committee on Professional Liability American Academy of Orthopaedic Surgeons 1996.
6. Richards P, Kennedy IM, Lord Woolf. Managing medical mishaps *BMJ* 1996; 313: 243–244.

Chapter

1

WHY DO PATIENTS SUE THEIR SURGEONS?

Every surgeon's heart misses a beat when they read the solicitors letter that a patient intends to sue them. Their thoughts begin to race. First, is it justified? Is it correct that they are guilty of some mismanagement, or has the patient misunderstood the situation? And secondly, why has this particular patient decided to sue? Perhaps the surgeon remembers that this complication has occurred before and it did not result in alleged negligence.

The notes are retrieved and carefully reviewed to assist the memory, and not infrequently a picture develops of the patient, not only their surgical problem and outcome, but their personality and perhaps their reasons for pursuing a claim. Doctors need to really understand why a patient is complaining if they are to satisfy them without further resource to the law, and also if they are to avoid the same problem in the future.

All surgeons make mistakes at some time during their career. They remember when they could have done better, when certain complications could have been avoided, and thankfully their patients did not seek redress. With regret it may be possible to identify times when a poor outcome resulted from a genuine mistake. And there was no resort to litigation, perhaps because communications were good. There was an explanation and an apology, and a good doctor–patient relationship meant that litigation was avoided.

A CHANGING SOCIETY

Claims of alleged negligence are steadily increasing and we have to ask what makes patients take this course. We are certainly living in a rapidly changing society. There is increasing expectation about outcome, standards of care and shared information. Patients are more willing to express disappointment when complications occur. They want to know if they have had a complication or an accident. If an accident, they look for a full explanation of what went wrong, and they may be angry. They need to know that it is not likely to happen to others. In a financially orientated society, angry patients look for compensation.

In addition, the surgeon can no longer take for granted the protection that comes from respect for professional authority. There was a time when the surgeon knew best, or (s)he thought (s)he did, and patients did as they were told. But now paternalism is dead, and everyone is considered accountable. Changing attitudes are largely responsible for the increase in allegations of negligence.

There are two important reasons why patients consider suing their surgeon:

(i)   they believe that there has been an accident, something went wrong. It should not normally happen, and they or their relative has been a victim;

(ii)   they claim that they were not forewarned. Even though they may not have had an accident, but rather they have suffered from a recognized complication that can occur in expert hands, they believe that they were either not forewarned or they were misinformed about the degree of risk. With foreknowledge they would not have had surgery.

Additional factors:

- lack of respect for the patient;
- unfulfilled expectations;
- the political climate;
- the patient's personality;
- criticism from colleagues;
- no explanation;
- no apology;
- anger.

These patients have a grievance, and now there is a choice to sue or not to sue. Let us look in detail at the many reasons for patients perusing a legal claim and what their alternative options are.

AN ACCIDENT

The patient may believe that, as a result of bad surgery, they are suffering from some complication that would not otherwise have occurred. No reasonable doctor would have operated like this. Perhaps they have a foot drop and think that a spinal nerve root was damaged during surgery. The patient and the doctor, and eventually the solicitor, will have to decide whether an accident occurred. If so, was it an acceptable complication that can occur from time to time even in expert hands, or would no responsible surgeon have injured this nerve?

MISINFORMATION

In addition, many patients who sue believe that they were not given the correct information. For example, they may be surprised by an unexpected complication such as cerebro-spinal fluid leaking from the wound with the need for secondary surgery to close a fistula. They cannot remember having been warned of this possibility. If they continue with chronic back pain they may think that the leaking cerebro-spinal fluid was responsible, and argue that they would not have had spinal surgery if they had been forewarned of this possible complication.

When an unexpected complication has occurred, the decision to sue the surgeon often depends on an interplay of several supplementary factors.

Lack of respect for the patient

Some patients will sue because they believe that their complication was handled insensitively. They were looking for an explanation but communications were poor. They felt that the surgeon was not interested. The problem was not explained, particularly in the early days. There were perhaps many different doctors and nurses looking after the patient, each giving conflicting explanations about the cause of the problem.

They feel that they were not respected. Often they received the first explanation from a junior doctor. No senior person took the time to sit down and discuss carefully why this complication had occurred, what was to be the management, and what was the expected outcome. Perhaps it was not discussed with the relatives who are often the driving force for litigation.

The surgeon may need support from colleagues, and it is good to anticipate the patient's request for a second opinion, whilst still keeping the doors of communication open. A second opinion assures the patient that their problem is being taken seriously, that they are respected.

To many patients, the hospital complaints procedure does not appear to be impartial. A useful feature of the civil system, much appreciated by the patient, is that if they proceed beyond the initial stages of litigation their case is reviewed by an independent unbiased expert, instructed by their solicitor. It is through the litigation process that they often feel they receive a satisfactory explanation. In contrast to the complaints procedure they will see the report, have access to the notes and they can discuss the case with their expert. If their suspicions are confirmed, there is relief that they were right to persist with their complaint. If, however, they have misunderstood the situation the expert can reassure them and clarify the position. This degree of respect at an earlier stage might prevent many legal proceedings.

Unfulfilled expectations

Surgeons may not be aware of the patient's and relatives' expectations. They are sometimes unreasonable. The right to health care may be misinterpreted by the patient as a right to be healthy. This is fuelled both by the media, and by a false understanding of science. In the real world, unfortunately, there are times when disease and disability can neither be avoided nor successfully treated, and patients who have unrealistic expectations will be severely disappointed. In this climate, surgeons need to spend more time explaining that an operation will not always produce full health and function.

A realistic explanation of outcome

Especially in spinal surgery, the patient needs a realistic explanation about the expected outcome. At best, they can hope for improvement. Only rarely will surgery produce a completely pain-free spine. If patients do not understand this at the outset, they may eventually sue their surgeon because they failed to make a full recovery. It is dangerous to say to a patient that following a spinal operation they will recover fully, be back to work in 6 weeks, and soon playing sport again. This can be the successful outcome, but it is never guaranteed.

Junior doctors do not usually have enough knowledge to appreciate the probable outcome from spinal surgery, and they should explain this to the patients. It is therefore the consultant's responsibility to give this information [1]. When the process of obtaining informed consent has been meticulously followed with adequate documentation (see Chapter 3), the truly informed patient can be neither surprised nor angry when spinal surgery has a less than perfect result.

Day-to-day management

Patients also expect that information about their day-to-day management and progress will be shared with them and their relatives. This has always been good practice. Patients expect it and it is due to them. Failure to communicate with the patient about their on-going treatment is rarely sufficient grounds for litigation, but it does breed resentment, and when things go wrong it is frequently the catalyst for allegations of negligence. A chain of minor errors may cascade into a major mishap.

It has always been good practice for the consultant who did the operation to visit the patient frequently in the post-operative days. The patient is examined and progress is discussed. A junior doctor makes clinical notes on progress every day. The patient is given an explanation about the reasons for ancillary tests with feedback about the results. There are discussions with the patient and relatives about what was found and done at the operation, about subsequent progress and about any complications. The doctors, nursing staff and physiotherapists are seen to be working as a team. On discharge there is clear advice about the after-care and rehabilitation, and a discharge summary is sent promptly to the general practitioner. A reasonable patient expects this good practice and, when adopted, it will compensate for the occasional error.

It is a patient's right to expect that their life and health will be protected to an acceptable professional standard. Legally accepted practice is that which a responsible body of medical opinion would deem appropriate in the clinical circumstances in which that practice occurs. This, however, is the minimum, and every doctor aims at the highest standard of care, particularly in regard to shared information.

The political climate

Political comment and media presentations on the health service have a powerful effect on public opinion. Adverse criticism undermines the nation's confidence in health care. Responsible leaders should think twice before gaining cheap advantage by unjustly criticizing hospitals and doctors. There is an expensive spin-off. Excessive media coverage about occasional poor standards makes the public critical of hospital care and individuals conscious of litigation.

It is ironic that opposition parties find political advantage in destroying the credibility of those seeking to provide a good health service. When in power, these same people ask how they can reduce the costs of litigation.

The patient's personality

Little has been written about the psychology of patients who sue their doctors, but those surgeons who have a medico-legal practice recognize that the personality of the patient can be important. The history may reveal that there has been unhappiness with the medical profession, sometimes a whole series of grievances and a previous attempt at litigation. Some of these patients often have a lack of self-worth, and problems in building up and maintaining relationships. It would be an injustice to suggest that this is a common feature of litigants, but there is a substantial minority who have personality problems which seem to antedate the claim. These patients are also prone to develop abnormal pain behaviour, with a non-organic component added to the disability.

Patients who exhibit abnormal pain behaviour are at risk of having a poor operative result, irrespective of the organic pathology (see Chapter 13). Non-organic features are not a contra-indication to surgery if there is a symptomatic pathology that can be corrected by operation. The organic component may be causing anxiety and distress, which can respond to expeditious surgery. However, the surgeon is alert to the possibility that distress may continue post-operatively, and could contribute to dissatisfaction.

Criticism from colleagues

Doctors, nurses and para-medical staff should refrain from unjust criticism of colleagues. This can be the origin of many litigation problems which are subsequently found to be groundless. One rarely knows all the facts and, when asked for an official or unofficial second opinion, it is important to be circumspect until all the evidence is available. Hasty verbal criticism can sow the seeds of suspicion in the patient's mind, and adverse written comments can have serious consequences that may subsequently be regretted (see Chapter 2).

The response of the medical profession

A satisfactory explanation

The patient's prime concern is for a satisfactory explanation about what went wrong, and for investigations to confirm it. Many patients sue simply because this explanation was denied them. Only 15% of litigants believe that they were given a satisfactory explanation for what went wrong [2]. In addition, they say that motivation for litigation was determined by the way the original incident was handled by the staff in the days or weeks following the accident. Most patients and relatives who sue believe that the sub-standard care extended well beyond the time of the original mishap, both in the ward and thereafter, and attitudes tend to harden. This would suggest that the doctor and staff concerned should sit down at an early stage with the patient and relatives and offer them a full explanation. Unfortunately, once there is a suggestion of recourse to the law, the common response is to close ranks and withdraw the lines of communication.

A changed practice

Complaints procedures are available, but in spite of attempts to make them more accessible to patients, they are still slow and complex, and often frustrating and bewildering [3]. Patients become angry because they find the process seldom leads to any real assurance that changes will be made to clinical practice.

Failure to apologize

An important objective of potential litigants is to receive an apology. Unfortunately doctors, if not culpable, feel vulnerable and threatened and tend to react defensively when things go wrong. They are perceived as being reluctant to apologize. Medical defence societies used to encourage their members to react like motorists involved in an accident and admit no liability. Fortunately this policy has changed. Without a frank and sympathetic explanation accompanied by a timely expression of regret or an apology, a relationship of trust disintegrates into an adversarial contest between embattled doctors and bruised families [2].

It should not be difficult for doctors to express regret when complications occur. This is what patients and relatives want to hear. It is not necessary to admit liability. They want to know that the surgeon is genuinely sorry, and they need to hear an expression of sympathy.

Case Report 1: Sympathy and regret on the fifth post-operative day. "I am so sorry Mrs J that you have this unpleasant pain in your leg. We think a nerve must have been bruised at the time of the operation. Sometimes when removing a disc protrusion, even very gentle retraction on the nerve can affect its blood supply and cause this type of pain and weakness after surgery. It means that the nerve was almost damaged before we started. It does not often happen. In fact I can only remember one other patient of mine like this. Fortunately he made a good recovery. I think it is likely that your pain will slowly settle down in the next 10 days, and that the strength will return to your foot maybe in 4 to 6 weeks. However, I am going to arrange for an MRI scan today to be sure that there is not another piece of disc pressing on the nerve. If that were the case we would want to operate again quite quickly, but I doubt if that is the case. The chances are that this is the result of a bruised nerve and it will slowly get better."

Six weeks later when Mrs J was no better. "I know just how distressing it is for you to still have this unpleasant pain, and still your foot is very weak. I hope the foot appliance is helping you to walk better, and that the medication is helping you to sleep at night. I am so sorry that there is still so little progress. As you know the MRI scan did not show any obvious problem, but I am arranging for Mr S to come and see you tomorrow to confirm that we are doing the right thing for you and that we have not missed anything. Quite frankly I still think it is the result of a bruised nerve, and I would not give up hope of a full recovery if we give it time. You know I am always available to talk to you and any other members of your family if it will help."

Three months later when there was still no improvement. "Mrs J what can I say to you! I am really sorry to see you like this. It is a great disappointment for me, when I had hoped you would have been almost fully recovered and back to work by now. Yes, when we discussed the operation with you, we did expect a good result. I would generally be discharging you by now. You are correct that we did not discuss the specific risk of a dropped foot, but I explained to you and to Mr J on more than one occasion that there are always a few patients who do not do well, and in fact can be worse after surgery. I did record this in my notes and in a letter to your GP – that there is a small risk of the nerve pain continuing, and there is a risk of a few people being worse after surgery with pain and some weakness. I know you did not expect to be one of these few people with a poor result, and I am truly sorry it is you. Mr S agrees with me that there is no need for any further surgery. However, you know we will continue to do all we can for you. I want you to see our Pain Specialist, and I will continue to see you every few months until we see some improvement."

It is usually the attitude of the doctor that will determine whether or not a patient will consider litigation. An explanation, and expressions of sympathy and sorrow will frequently satisfy a disappointed patient. "A gentle answer turns away wrath" [4]. However, some patients had higher expectations, they are angry and so convinced that there has been a serious mistake that they will not be pacified. They do not believe that the explanations that are offered are true, and they think expressions of sympathy are merely a sham, a smoke screen to cover serious mismanagement.

Anger

Patients who sue their doctors are often angry. They are either angry that the surgeon has made a serious mistake, or that they were not given the correct information prior to surgery. Sometimes no amount of time and explanation will satisfy them. These patients want justice and redress. Someone must be accountable and must pay either in monetary terms or by suffering.

Patients also expect that a system will be introduced to see that this problem is not repeated, that it does not happen to another patient. Where appropriate, patients should be told about the changes that have been made to prevent future incidents – altering systems or education of staff. The *Daily Telegraph* reported that relatives of a patient who died under anaesthetic said "If she was killed by a doctor's negligence, then we want justice and we want to make sure that no one else has to go through the pain that we have suffered" [5].

Vincent *et al.* [6] identified four main reasons why people who have a poor outcome may sue their doctors:

(i) concern with standards of care;

(ii) the need for an explanation;

(iii) the desire for compensation;

(iv) the belief that medical staff are accountable.

A feeling of anger was the main emotion in 90% of patients who sued their doctor. Bitterness was described by 80%, betrayal by 55% and 40% had strong feelings of humiliation (see *Table 1.1*).

Anger is believed to be justified when the patient feels that they are not treated with respect. It is more common when they have unrealistic expectations, and if they have an aggressive personality. It is fuelled by criticism (just or unjust) from medical colleagues.

Legal disputes cannot always be avoided, especially if there is a serious mishap or a very angry patient. However, as doctors try to develop a greater spirit of candour, humility and partnership with their patients, claimants may be encouraged to use the internal complaints procedures, mediation and other informal means of resolution [2]. At the present time, the average time to judgement in claims for compensation is 5–7 years [7]. Surgeons and managers should be working to prevent litigation and, when it is inevitable, for both parties to make realistic offers to settle at the earliest possible stage – a faster, cheaper and less painful process than the current lengthy litigation procedure which causes so much distress.

Table 1.1 Ranking of reasons for litigation

Doctor's perception	Patient's perception
1. Retribution	1. Honesty/explanation/apology
2. Compensation	2. Avoid repetition
3. Avoid repetition	3. Compensation
4. Honesty/explanation/apology	4. Retribution

REFERENCES

1. Soin B, Thompson H, Smellie W. Informed consent: A case for more education of the surgical team. *Ann. R. Coll. Surg. Engl.* 1993; 75: 62–65.
2. Richards P, Kennedy IM, Lord Woolf. Managing medical mishaps. *BMJ* 1996; 313: 243–244.
3. Donaldson LJ, Cavenagh JJ. Clinical complaints and their handling: a time for change. *Qual. Health Care* 1992; 1: 21.
4. *The Bible*. Proverbs chapter 15, verse 1.
5. The *Daily Telegraph*, 30 December 1997.
6. Vincent C, Young M, Phillips A. Why do people sue their doctors? A study of patients and relatives taking legal action. *The Lancet* 1994; 343: 1609–1611.
7. Bowden MF. Compensation should be analogous to prompt payment of a bill. *BMJ* 1998; 316: 74.

Chapter
2

THE LEGAL PROCESS AND PROBLEMS

PROOF OF MEDICAL NEGLIGENCE

The solicitor who instructs an expert witness wants to know three things:

(i)   whether there would be a body of responsible clinicians who would have treated that patient in that manner;

(ii) whether there has been an injury;

(iii) what are the consequences.

Minimally competent doctor

The Bolam case has established that in English and Welsh law at the present time, the plaintiff must be able to show that no responsible body of clinicians would have treated them in this manner [1]. A doctor "is not guilty of negligence if he has acted in accordance with a practice accepted as proper". Similarly it has been said that "the true test for establishing liability in diagnosis or treatment on the part of a Doctor is whether or not he has been proved to be guilty of such failure as no Doctor of ordinary skill and care would be guilty of" [2]. The standard expected is that adopted at the time of the injury and not in present-day practice. The expected skills in that particular hospital and by that grade of doctor are also relevant.

The burden of proof is not on the defendant but on the plaintiff to show that they believe there has been negligence. The facts are medical and not legal, and hence the plaintiff relies heavily on the opinion of the medical expert.

An injury

When the law is considering personal injury there is usually no doubt that an injury has occurred. In medical negligence, however, there may be uncertainty about an injury, and it has to be proved. When deciding what happened, and the outcome, the court is interested in the balance of probabilities – 'is it more likely than not' – sometimes expressed as more than 51% – which is a lesser standard than that adopted by doctors in their normal practice. Certainty or near certainty is not required.

The outcome

The plaintiff has to show that as a consequence of injury there has been an unfavourable outcome. This, again, may not be easy to establish when one considers the probable natural history.

THE MEDICAL REPORT

Courts repeatedly stress that the role of the expert is to be impartial. Although instructed by one side, the medical opinion cannot be tailored to support that side's case.

Acceptable standard

When providing a medical report about injury, outcome and minimal competence, the expert witness does not have the remit to say that there has been negligence. That is for the judge to decide, or for the defence to admit.

The solicitor requests an expert opinion, and the first report is not usually for disclosure. The doctor is free to express any difficulties that might be anticipated in pursuing or defending this claim. The report should assist the solicitor, and subsequently the barrister, to decide whether or not there is a likely case of negligence.

Outcome

It is helpful to the lawyers assessing the potential of a claim if the doctor providing the first report can also describe what the adverse results of poor practice are. The expert witness may then be asked to clarify certain aspects of the report, and the report for the plaintiff's solicitors is discussed with the plaintiff.

Condition and prognosis

When proceedings are issued it is necessary to serve a 'Condition and Prognosis' report. The expert witness may be requested to examine the plaintiff and provide this second report. Reference can be made to the medical notes and the investigations, but not to the plaintiff's statement which is a privileged document. There should be no comments about liability and causation in this report.

Plaintiff satisfaction

It is essential that the plaintiff understands and is satisfied with the report(s). Perhaps for the first time they appreciate that there has not been an injury, or that any injury has not had an adverse outcome. They may now understand that they have suffered a complication that can unfortunately occur even in skilful hands, and the claim goes no further. Alternatively there is need for a conference.

A CONFERENCE

The plaintiff often has preconceived ideas that have become entrenched over 2 or 3 years. They may not agree with the medical report(s). A conference with the barrister, solicitor, expert witness, plaintiff and a friend can be very helpful. It should enable the plaintiff to understand what the legal requirements to establish medical negligence are. They will have the opportunity to see the barrister question the expert witness and establish that the opinion is reasonable. It also gives the plaintiff the chance to talk to the expert witness, expressing their concerns and perhaps misunderstandings. The plaintiff is the most important person at the conference, and at the close they should feel that they have been given good advice and are being properly represented.

PLEADING

If the barrister or solicitor considers that there is a reasonable claim for negligence, a pleading will be written, and the expert witness may be asked to confirm the accuracy of the medical facts. This is then presented to the defence, who reply. There may follow an amended pleading from the plaintiff, and requests from either side for better and further particulars of either pleading, requests for interrogatories or notices to admit. The expert will probably be required in these various stages to scrutinize suggested requests and replies.

TIMESCALE

In English and Welsh law, the defence has 3 years from the time of knowledge in which to submit a claim for medical negligence. It may be many months before a patient seeks legal advice, because it takes the health service an average of 9 months to investigate complaints. One hospital trust was described as being "inflexible, bureaucratic and unhelpful". Although it is in the interest of all parties to speed up the legal process, solicitors have difficulty in retrieving medical records and then instructing doctors to provide reports. Unless they are efficiently represented, plaintiffs may run out of time.

PROBLEMS FOR THE DEFENCE

Doctors fear being in court to defend their professional reputation. Even if they are shown to be innocent, the publicity involved is very traumatic and it leaves a scar for a lifetime. Understandably, their representatives attempt to settle any reasonable case out of court, away from the glare of the media. In some areas of uncertainty, when the court's probable decision is uncertain, in order to protect the doctor the defence may agree to the plaintiff's allegations.

There are a number of specific factors that can interfere with the successful defence of claims, particularly if there has been poor documentation and criticism from other colleagues. Surgeons who wish to protect themselves should be aware of these difficulties.

Medical records

When the legal process begins, the first task is to retrieve and examine the medical records. These records are the principle weapon in defending any claim of negligence. The medical notes may be a disappointment, causing serious problems for the defence. The surgeon may be innocent, but an adequate defence may be difficult if it is not supported by the records. They are sometimes of such poor quality that they do not substantiate the surgeon's claim. In addition, they may contain incriminating evidence from colleagues, albeit unjust, of poor practice. Good clinical record-keeping and caution when providing a second opinion might have resulted in a different legal outcome. However, sloppy practice in documentation and unsubstantiated opinions can condemn a surgeon even though (s)he may be innocent of negligence. These are lessons for every surgeon.

Complete records

Medical records should document the actual events as treatment progresses. They should also reflect the doctor's ongoing assessment of each problem and management plan. In addition, the thought process when considering each problem and deciding on a course of action should be clearly documented. The courts are often unwilling to find fault with doctors for scientific error if the reasons for management are clearly stated, because there is usually more than one 'right way' to deal with a given problem.

First attendance
It is good practice when the patient first attends to record a complete history – the onset of pain, its site, duration, periodicity, with aggravating and relieving factors and overall disability. The patient is usually taken through a normal day noting the effects of standing, sitting, walking, work and recreation. Previous investigations and therapies are noted with their effects. There needs to be a record of a full clinical examination of the spine, and lower limbs. A differential diagnosis is noted, with plans for investigations and possible management.

Second visit
On the second visit there should be a record of the surgeon's interpretation of the investigations, and that the surgeon has seen the results of these investigations and the X-rays. There needs to be a careful description of what was said to the patient about management options. If surgery was discussed, then the risks and benefits of an operation should be written down, and how this compares with conservative management and with the natural history. The patient's views also need to be recorded. It is helpful if this information is in the clinical notes, and is summarized again in a letter to the general practitioner after each visit.

Further visits
It is good practice to see the patient on a further occasion before deciding on surgery. This gives the patient an opportunity to reconsider the management plan, and allows the surgeon to describe again the risks and benefits of various options. Only then can the surgeon be confident that the patient really understands the issues, and that there is genuine shared decision making.

The operation
This should be described in the notes in detail. If there are any unusual or unexpected findings they should be recorded. Any complications should be carefully noted. For example, if the dura was accidentally torn, the site and extent of the damage should be noted and how it was managed.

The defence lawyers will appreciate detailed operation notes, rather than a brief, three line, nondescript record, even though the surgeon knows that the operation was a routine procedure. In a court of law, brief handwritten operation notes may suggest a casual approach to the operation, and give a poor impression. Comprehensive typewritten notes will support the view that the surgeon was also careful and meticulous in the operative procedure. It is common practice to write the details of the operation by hand immediately after the procedure, and for the secretary to transcribe these notes the following day.

Post-operative care
One of the duties of the consultant surgeon is to train the junior doctors to maintain good quality and regular post-operative records. This is supplemented by occasional notes by the surgeon who did the operation. Most surgeons record only positive signs, and if the patient is progressing well, it is sufficient to simply record this good progress. The absence of extensive post-operative notes usually means that the patient is progressing well, but a daily note to that effect is good practice. However, complications are carefully noted, as well as what is said to the patient about any adverse problems. If there are serious complications, the operating surgeon needs to write down what is the probable cause, what investigations are to be carried out and a proposed method of management.

It is important that the notes are legible, consecutive and preferably typewritten. Such comprehensive records suggest good overall practice. It has to be admitted, however, that there is a body of responsible surgeons who, through pressure of work and substandard support facilities, are unable to maintain this high standard.

Accurate records

Accuracy
No one can avoid error from time to time, but inaccuracy in the medical records is unhelpful to the defence. For example, one expects to see accuracy and consistency about the dates of various events, the side of the symptoms,

the segmental level of the operation and the operative procedure. Accuracy in recording is compatible with the truth about what is claimed to have been said to the patient.

Timing of knowledge of error

When a genuine mistake has been made, such as operating at the wrong level or the wrong side, the surgeon should write this in the records and the time the error was first noted, with an explanation of what was said to the patient. An honest admission of error is always preferred by the defending lawyers, than blank notes. Failure to record can appear as a devious cover up.

Offensive comments

It is important that medical records are free of comments that might be considered offensive to those who may subsequently read them. Derogatory statements about the patient or any other physician should be carefully avoided. This practice is taught in medical schools, but it is not always appreciated by older surgeons.

Changing records

Altering the records at a later date is unforgivable. Medical notes that have been changed after the fact provide perfect ammunition to immediately settle a claim in favour of the plaintiff. Whatever high quality care has been provided to the patient, an altered record makes a case indefensible. The courts tend not to believe doctors who alter records. Erasure and white outs, and notes added to the margin to clarify earlier entries are absolutely contraindicated.

The surgeon should use great caution if a change in the record is needed. If there is a change of view about what happened, then it is reasonable to record this altered view at a later date, with an appropriate explanation. There may be need for amplification or an explanatory amendment at the end of the record, but this should include the current date, and why the information was added at that time.

Contemporary records

When very serious complications occur, there can be an emergency situation where record keeping takes second place to immediate management. However, an accurate record of the timing of the events and of remedial action can be crucial for the defence. Even though the overriding priority is to diagnose and treat an unexpected emergency, and keeping notes takes second place, at a later date if there is no good record which is accurately timed, the treating physicians will appear to be unprofessional. Conversely, good notes generated contemporaneously which monitor intervention and the patient's progress will convince the courts that the doctors were in control of a difficult situation.

Junior staff should have been trained to keep contemporary records during this type of clinical emergency, and it only takes a moment for the supervising surgeon to ensure that this is taking place. As soon as there is a moment of respite, it is high priority that the senior doctors should write their own notes.

Case Report 2: *No records!* JG seemed to have an uneventful operation to correct an adolescent idiopathic scoliosis, but in the recovery room it was noted that his blood pressure was only 50/30 and he had a tachycardia of 140 per minute. The wound was inspected and it was bleeding profusely. There was considerable panic as the anaesthetist called for more blood, and there was difficulty introducing a new intravenous line. It was not possible to find the surgeon who had done the operation because he had just left the theatre complex to visit the wards.

The team worked hard to maintain blood volume, and no contemporary notes were recorded for 3 hours. Only subsequently did the clinicians find time to record how the blood replacement had slowly re-established an acceptable blood pressure of 110/70 and pulse of 100 per minute.

Subsequently it was unclear how much intravenous fluid had been replaced and at what speed, and how quickly the circulation had been restored. In addition, there was no contemporary explanation as to when the surgeon had returned to theatre, nor why the surgeon did not choose to re-operate and remove a haematoma. The thinking process behind the management plan was not recorded. The boy developed neurological complications which were alleged to be due to a combination of 2 hours hypotension in association with a haematoma pressing on the spinal cord. The lack of contemporary notes was a problem for the defence.

Criticism from colleagues

Jousting
Sometimes claims of malpractice arise because of unjust criticism from colleagues. The criticism may be direct or implied. Clinicians should know the consequences of this 'jousting', which is extremely damaging to colleagues who may find themselves defending time-consuming, unjust allegations. One rarely knows all the facts. An ill-considered chance remark is often remembered by an unhappy patient, to become the germ of a litigation claim.

Case Report 3: *You should have come to see me sooner.* Miss JB was a 27-year-old secretary who had been troubled for 2 years with pain in the back which was referred to the right thigh. She had seen an eminent orthopaedic surgeon who, after an examination and X-ray, told her that although she had a back problem it did not require surgery. She heard of another surgeon who was carrying out chymopapain injections. He was very sympathetic, and he told her "You should have come to see me sooner". A MRI scan showed a mildly bulging disc at L4/5. It was not affecting the nerve root. Although the pain was more in her back than in the leg, it did not radiate below the knee and there were no root tension signs, he treated her with chymopapain. Not surprisingly, she was no better.

Three years later she was suing both her general practitioner and the first orthopaedic surgeon for delay in referral for chymopapain. She claimed, on the basis of a chance remark, that her long-term disability could have been avoided by earlier referral. The claim was unfair and it was not successful, but it's defence involved a great deal of time and expense.

Second opinion

When asked to provide a second opinion, spinal surgeons should have all the available data before giving a written view about a diagnosis, or the cause of a complication and its prognosis and management. It is necessary to review the complete inpatient and outpatient records and radiographs, scans and other investigations. The surgeon should also try to discuss the patient's prior care with the previously treating doctor, which will help to clarify all the aspects of care and the thought processes which led to that management. Only then is it possible to provide a reasonable opinion.

A clear and straightforward explanation can be a great help to a troubled patient. Many patients have had unreasonable expectations, and perhaps are now able to take a realistic view. There has been no accident or error, and there should be no unnecessary criticism. The doctor has not been asked to give a view on potential negligence. Furthermore, if a doctor does unreasonably criticize a colleague, and the patient is encouraged to take retributive action, the second doctor will often be named as a co-defendant in the legal action. Even when no injury and no negligence is found, the time and expense in defending against such a claim is usually considerable.

This cautious approach to criticism is not to deny the obligation doctors have to injured patients and to protect them against harmful or sick surgeons or dangerous environments, but this will be discussed in Chapter 19.

REFERENCES

1. Case of *Bolam* v. *Friern Hospital Management Committee* [1957] 2 All ER 118.
2. Hunter 1955 *SLT reference* 101.

Chapter
3

INFORMED CONSENT

We are living in a generation when patients are well informed about health. It is not unusual to meet a patient who has done a literature search, scanned the internet, made their own provisional diagnosis and knows what they want from their surgeon. Their understanding may be imperfect, they may have little knowledge of treatment options and outcome, but they already have some information and they want more [1]. They also want to be involved in making decisions about their management [2].

Patients believe that good information means "honest, unbiased, up to date information about their illness, its likely outcome and the risk and benefits of different interventions. They want help to identify and secure their treatment preferences. When uncertainty exists it should be discussed, not omitted or glossed over, and advice should be explicitly supported by the best available evidence" [3]. It is hardly surprising that when this information is denied them, and when things go wrong, patients are inclined to sue. The most common cause for patient dissatisfaction is not clinical competency but communication, a failure to receive sufficient information about the surgery and its risks [4].

At the present time surgeons agree that prior to surgery every patient must know the risks and benefits of the operation. But who is to tell them, how much should they be told, how can the informer be sure the patient understands, how long does it take and how should information be recorded? To what degree is it permissible for the surgeon to try to influence the patient's decision?

WHO SHOULD PROVIDE INFORMED CONSENT?

Establishing a good patient–doctor relationship is at the heart of real medicine. It is founded on mutual respect. The importance the surgeon gives to consent indicates his respect for the patient, and it cements the relationship. If they are given sufficient information, patients usually know better than anyone else what is good for them. They should be able to make their own decision provided it is based on information and support. They will then usually remain content, even if things go wrong.

The consultant is the best person to obtain this informed consent. Spinal surgery is major surgery and it is not good practice for the consultant to delegate discussions about a spinal operation to a trainee. It is the consultant who is responsible for the patient's management, and this means that the consultant should also discuss the option of surgery with the patient. There can be exceptions if one considers the seniority of the trainee and the type and the urgency of surgery.

There are only a few absolute indications for spine surgery – tumour, trauma, infection and a massive lesion in the spinal canal involving the bladder. Surgery for most other back pain problems is relative. It is a balance of risks and benefits. It takes mature judgement to relate this to each individual patient, and only after careful and frank discussion between the consultant and the patient, can the decision to operate become a shared and sensible decision.

HOW MUCH SHOULD THE PATIENT BE TOLD?

How much information?

Patients differ about how much they want to know about their medical condition, and when they want to know it. They should be given as much information as they need or desire. There is evidence, however, that patients want more information than they get, and that doctors overestimate how much they supply [5]. In the Bolam case, the law sets the level 'at the standard adopted by the medical profession'. A doctor giving as much information as would be offered by a recognized body of medical opinion at that time is not usually held liable in law [6].

However, doctors should be prepared to go further. Good practice is not the same as the legal minimum. Lord Scarman believes the standard amount of information given should be what the average 'prudent patient' would want to know [7]. Courts are now prepared to question very critically the 'responsible body of opinion' which is currently presented to support the defence.

Understanding information

Every patient should have an understanding of their condition. At the time of the first consultation they may already be well informed about their problem, having seen other doctors and therapists. At the outset, therefore, it is helpful to know what a patient already knows about their diagnosis. If they are asked about it, they will use their own words and the clinician can then use the same vocabulary to help in communication. One can add in greater detail what they do not already know, filling in gaps and correcting the misconceptions.

When explaining the diagnosis and various treatment options, including no treatment, it is helpful to use diagrams, drawings, models and to demonstrate the observed pathology on the X-rays and scans. Patients want a simple explanation in a language they can understand.

It is important that all doctors diagnosing and treating spinal disorders are honest and express uncertainty when that is present. Ignorance is common when dealing with chronic low back pain, and the surgeon frequently has to express uncertainty. Some patients cope better with this than others.

> **Case Report 4:** *Alcohol*. Mr JR attended the clinic smelling of alcohol. The surgeon could not really obtain a coherent history and, as he hesitated, JR asked what was the matter. "I don't know" the consultant said "it could be the drink". "Don't worry doctor" said JR "I quite understand, I'll come back and see you next week"!

Understanding the diagnosis

Junior doctors especially should be prepared to admit to patients that they have limited experience and they may know neither the diagnosis nor the prognosis. They will protect themselves if they request help from a more senior surgeon. They learn as they listen to their consultants discuss the diagnosis, and the risks and benefits of surgery.

> **Case Report 5:** *What is the diagnosis?* Mr HK was a 52-year-old ex-miner. He had had 6 years of increasing problems with his lower back until he could work no longer. Clinical examination and investigations by MRI and discogram suggested that the L4/5 segment was pathological and a possible pain source. He wanted to know if surgery could help him.
>
> "The good news Mr K is that I think we can localize the problem. The investigations suggest that the pain is coming from one of the lower segments of the lumbar spine, at L4/5. The disc is rather worn and degenerate, and the little joints at the back, the facet joints, are also rather worn. Let me draw a diagram. This disc has been getting degenerate for many years, probably even before you ever experienced your first pain. It is something that often happens without any injury. All the other discs look good. Let me show you the X-rays. Now we can't be totally sure that your pain is coming from this segment, though I think it is the most likely diagnosis. Now please stop me if you don't understand what I am saying."
>
> "You had a discogram at the previous hospital, and I have a letter here that says the injection into this disc reproduced your pain. However, one can not always be confident about this test, although it does support the diagnosis that the L4/5 segment is causing some pain. No one can really tell you which part of this segment is causing the pain. It might be the

edge of the disc, or the bone being sensitive adjacent to the disc. Another possibility is that the small facet joints are painful, or it may be the ligaments and the muscles getting strained and fatigued when you do too much. All we can say is that some part of this segment is probably responsible for your pain."

Understanding the prognosis

It is important to be honest about the prognosis. Some patients have to come to terms with chronic back pain, and need to know that they are likely to continue with some pain and disability.

> **Continuing Case Report 5 of Mr HK**. *What is the prognosis?* "You are asking if I can give you a second opinion about an operation. Well let's talk first about how things are likely to go without an operation. I think it is very likely the symptoms will not change very much. You have retired, and are putting less strain on your back, but having had this pain for 10 years, it is likely to go on troubling you. I don't think it will get any worse, but you are likely to continue with pain when you walk a long way and you are not going to be able to do those car repairs, DIY and gardening that you enjoyed a few years ago. And there are no more simple therapies that will change things. You have had quite energetic rehabilitation, and a spell at the pain clinic. If you don't have surgery, then I think the best thing is to keep as fit as possible and accept the problem. It will not change much."

Understanding the risks and benefits of surgery

Doctors do not always agree about the natural history of a condition nor about the risks of certain procedures. Relevant information in the literature may be based on highly selected groups of patients, which bears little resemblance to the particular patient in front of them [8]. Research literature may be of poor quality or irrelevant to ordinary clinical practice. Statistical probabilities may mean little to that surgeon or to that individual patient. And steering one's way through the evidence jungle takes time, skill and perseverance.

Furthermore, one surgeon's complication rate may differ from that of another. There is an inequality of health care, and it is difficult to measure how great this is. Up to the present time surgeons have not conducted a continuous audit of their performance. There are difficulties because the young surgeon has a learning curve, and complication rates will vary with experience. Risks are therefore usually presented in broad terms.

However, patients have the right to ask their hospital doctor for increasingly comprehensive information on the success rates of their unit's procedures compared with national figures. Knowing about these risks is a prerequisite for patients to exercise their common law right to give informed consent.

The minimum information due to a patient about surgical management is

- what are the broad benefits of surgery in the short and long term – what is the chance of improvement, and how much improvement
- what are the risks of remaining the same
- what is the risk of being worse
- how does this compare with the natural history in the short and long term
- how does this hospital unit compare with the national average.

For many patients this is all they want to know, and if described in percentage terms as realistically as possible for that unit and for that surgeon, this may be enough information for them to make a rational decision.

Continuing Case Report 5 of Mr HK. *What are the surgical risks and benefits?* "Mr J has told you that there is a 60% chance of success with a spinal fusion. I think that is correct. That means 60% chance of being improved, but really the chances of being quite free of pain, and able to do everything you did before, are not good. Most people with a good result of fusion feel a lot better, but they still have occasional pain, and have to be careful with their back. There is of course a chance (perhaps 30%) that you will be no better. The pain could continue as it is, in spite of a good fusion. That is because the pain may be coming from another segment, even though the other parts of your spine seem good on the various tests. Also, even in the best hands, an operation to fuse a segment may fail to fuse, and a degree of movement may continue to give some pain. Mr J also told you that there was a chance that you could be worse after surgery. That is correct. I would estimate that there is a 10% chance you could be worse, either with more back pain or because of some unexpected complication that can happen from time to time. You must not forget that with this type of surgery there is a chance that you could be worse."

"You ask me how things could be much worse? Well there is a chance of something happening like a nerve being damaged. That could give you some leg pain and some weakness. It does not often happen, perhaps in one or two in every hundred fusions. Very rarely many nerves are affected, giving water-work problems. I have to say occasionally the membrane around the nerves can be damaged and cause a leak of spinal fluid for a while. Occasionally it means a second operation. Rarely, wounds get infected, and there are occasional anaesthetic risks, and it is possible to get clots in the leg veins which affect the lungs."

"The last thing I want to do is frighten you. Most patients do well, and there is a better than 50/50 chance that you will be improved. However, you have to realize that a good result can not be guaranteed and, from time to time, patients are worse after a fusion."

"Now I want to be sure that you have understood what I have been saying. It is not easy to take in all this information at once. So would you mind telling me in your own words the main points I have been sharing with you."

"Yes you've got it exactly right. Do you have any more questions? I wonder if there is any underlying worry that you have not mentioned. Yes, I can confirm there is nothing at all to suggest that you have a tumour or anything serious."

"You tell me that you would like to give more thought to an operation but probably go ahead eventually. That makes good sense. I will write a letter to Mr J – whom I understand told you the same things – and I know if you want surgery, he will do his best for you. I will also write a letter to your GP. I think you should discuss these things with your GP and again with Mr J. I hope if you have a fusion you will be one of his successes."

Understanding the degree of risk

There are some spinal problems where the surgeon can be reasonably confident about a good result, but it is still important to respect the patient's autonomy, and not over-persuade them to have an operation. Spinal surgery is a life-threatening procedure for what is usually a non-life-threatening condition. Most patients do very well with surgery for disc protrusion, but they need to be fully aware of the occasional risks. A surgeon who neglects to discuss these complications will eventually face claims of medical negligence.

Case Report 6: *Benefits of disc surgery.* Mrs SJ was a 26-year-old teacher. She had had 8 weeks of sciatic pain from a disc protrusion, and could not work because of leg pain. She was told that surgery removing the disc fragment will dramatically relieve the leg pain in 90% of patients. There was about 10% chance of the leg pain remaining, not because the fragment is not effectively removed, but because the nerve can remain bruised, and may take time to recover. There was a remote chance of being worse – about 2–4% – because of some unforeseen problem common to all spine surgery, such as nerve damage, infection or anaesthetic risk. She was told the surgery will not influence her back ache and that 65% of patients continue with some back pain, varying in degree. Disc surgery is for leg pain not back pain. She asked if she could know more about the risks of being worse.

If this lady had agreed to surgery asking no further questions, it would have been reasonable for the consent form to be signed and to proceed. Too much discussion about risks is not justified. It can frighten a patient unnecessarily. However, when she requested more information the surgeon explained in more detail.

Continuing Case Report 6. *Risks of disc surgery.* The surgeon explained that during surgery a nerve root is occasionally damaged even in the best hands (two per hundred). This might cause a foot drop, even permanent foot weakness. On very rare occasions (three per thousand) the nerves to the bladder are damaged, and this is a disaster. Sometimes the membrane containing the spinal fluid is torn, causing a leak through the wound after surgery. The wound can get infected. Some patients get clots in the leg veins after surgery, and subsequent chest problems (less than one per hundred). She accepted these risks and agreed to surgery.

Every operation carries a small risk of mortality. When removing a disc there is a risk of perhaps one in 20 000 of injuring the great vessels of the aorta or inferior vena cava, and some of these patients will die. Should every patient be told of this life-threatening complication? In 1992 a court in Australia upheld a 'failure to warn' charge even though the risk was one in 14 000 (*Rogers v Whittaker*) [9]. This was because the damage – blindness in the one good eye – was so devastating. Many spine surgeons would argue that to describe such remote, though serious, risks engenders unacceptable fears in their patients. Provided they have explained that this type of surgery carries very occasional though serious risks, they believe that without being specific they have done their duty.

Lord Templeton has summed up the situation "A patient may make an unbalanced judgement because he is deprived of information. A patient may also make an unbalanced judgement if he is provided with too much information and is made aware of possibilities which he is not capable of assessing because of his lack of medical training, his prejudices, or his personality" [10].

> ***Continuing Case Report 6.*** *Unexpected neurological deficit.* When Mrs SJ recovered from what was thought to be an uneventful disc operation, she could neither feel nor move her legs. The surgeon who performed the operation saw her 2 hours after surgery, and noted that the sensation in her legs was 'patchy'. Peri-anal sensation was impaired. An emergency MRI scan was compatible with further extrusion of disc material. She had a second operation that evening, and only a small amount of further disc material was removed. A bony decompression was carried out because there was a degree of spinal stenosis. After surgery the nerve roots were thought to be free and not compressed. Unfortunately, this lady was left with a permanent bladder problem, poor sensation and weakness in her legs.
>
> She claimed that because the bladder nerves were permanently damaged, her surgeon must have operated negligently. She also said she could not remember her surgeon warning her of this specific risk to the bladder. However, this risk had been recorded in the notes, and on the issue of informed consent, the surgeon was exonerated.

HOW CAN WE BE SURE THAT THE PATIENT REALLY UNDERSTANDS?

This is a difficult question to answer. Firstly, some patients have little understanding of percentage risk. When considering surgery for a non-life-threatening condition, they may readily accept a 1% risk of dying under anaesthetic. However, the same person would think twice if told there was a one in a hundred chance of being knocked down crossing the road, and what does 1% mean if you are that person affected?

Secondly, it is also difficult to explain to a patient what each complication means in terms of disability. Because of psycho-social factors, every patient responds differently to a disability.

Thirdly, patients who are anxious with acute or chronic pain may find it difficult to comprehend that with time the pain will naturally resolve. They may not take in all the information at once. It helps to check that the information has been understood.

If the surgeon thinks that there is some doubt about what is really understood, the patient can be invited 'in their own words' to summarize the main issues. There is then an opportunity to correct any misunderstanding and repeat some of what was said. Patients often appreciate the chance to verbalize the situation. In the process they recognize that the doctor is trying to help, and that they are respected as a person. It also helps to establish a trusting relationship.

Doctors know that patients remember only a small part of the information they are given during a single consultation. They can misinterpret facts. Not infrequently patients say that they were told they would never walk again if they did not have surgery! It is not surprising, therefore, that some may complain that they were not told about any complications, even though a surgeon is adamant that it is always his practice to discuss these problems. It is unwise to assume that a patient understands, simply because they have been given verbal information.

Non-English-speaking patients will have particular difficulty appreciating the implications of surgery, and they must be given special care, usually with the help of a family friend or a trained interpreter.

Children under 16 years of age are not allowed to give consent to operation. In spinal surgery this is relevant when surgery is being carried out for a juvenile disc protrusion or for deformity. If a patient under 18 years of age refuses surgery, the Family Law Reform Act 1969 does not deprive parents of their right to authorize medical treatment if they believe it is in their child's interest [11].

HOW LONG DOES IT TAKE TO OBTAIN 'INFORMED CONSENT'?

Patients generally need time to come to a rational decision about spinal surgery. In some cultures they are invited to take home a video which describes the operation. They then return to the hospital at a later time with their decision. However, because of individual variations in pathology and personality, no video describes exactly the real-life situation for every patient.

There is probably no substitute for a good consultation which is unhurried, and is repeated on a second occasion before reaching a final, shared decision. This is time well spent. It not only ensures that information is shared and understood, but it builds up a good relationship, invaluable to both patient and doctor if there are unexpected complications.

HOW SHOULD THE INFORMATION BE RECORDED?

Hospital notes

Documentation of consent should usually be recorded by the consultant or senior surgeon who is going to perform the operation. It is good practice for the contemporaneous notes and a letter to the general practitioner to record

- what was said by the surgeon about risks and benefits at the consultation,
- to whom,
- what was the response of the patient and relative(s).

The consent form

The detailed recording of informed consent is much more than the signing of a consent form. The consent form was originally introduced to protect surgeons from the allegation of assault by patients who regretted the surgical intervention. This is still its important function. It is seen as a contract, concluding previous discussions about the operation, and it also has clinical value. An eminent judge recorded "The clinical purpose (*of consent forms*) stems from the fact that in many instances the co-operation of the patient and the patient's faith or at least confidence in the efficacy of the treatment is a major factor contributing to the treatment's success" [12].

This surgical consent form must be signed by patient and doctor just prior to the operation, and it is the house surgeon who usually obtains this written consent. It is good practice for the doctor issuing the consent form to leave this for the patient to read before it is signed, and to return later to collect the form. However, this alone is insufficient to establish that the patient understands the procedure and its risks. The junior doctor who usually signs this form is least qualified to give the correct information. Junior doctors often lack sufficient knowledge to fully inform patients and thus meet the legal requirements [13]. Rather, the facts about surgery should have been discussed by a senior surgeon when the patient's name was placed on the waiting list.

It is salutary that in a recent survey of junior doctors, only 27% knew that signing a consent form was not an end in itself, but rather the conclusion of previous discussions, and that complications should have been previously discussed and recorded. Many denied having any formal training about the use of consent forms [14].

The signing of the consent form should establish that the patient has understood the previous information discussed in the clinic. It is evidence of a process, not the process itself. The consultant who discussed the merits of surgery is the one who should already have recorded what was discussed, and this should have been in as much detail as possible. The evidence of this record means that the surgeon took the responsibility about informed consent seriously. The consent form establishes that no new events have changed that decision.

TO WHAT DEGREE IS IT PERMISSIBLE TO INFLUENCE THE PATIENT'S DECISION?

The days have long passed since the surgeon knew what was in the patient's best interest, and was the sole decision maker. However, some patients still stop the consultant and ask "What would you advise, doctor". Their final choice is to let the doctor choose. They find too much information confusing, and want the surgeon to make the decision. Most surgeons appreciate this and take their cue from the patient about how much information they can accept at any stage in their management.

There are also times when the surgeon feels the patient is making the wrong decision. In non-life-threatening conditions it is rarely justified to recommend surgery too strongly. However, it may be reasonable to slant the discussion to advise them not to have surgery. They may be anxious for an operation when this is not in their best interests.

> **Case Report 7:** *Wrong advice?* Mr HD was a 56-year-old farmworker. He had an isthmic spondylolisthesis which was thought to be responsible for 10 years of mild back pain, and increasing pain in the previous year. He had given up his job. Surgeon 'A' had suggested a spinal fusion, and he was keen to have surgery. Surgeon 'B' agreed that an operation would probably give 70% change of marked relief of pain, but thought conservative management had not been exhausted. He advised the patient to lose weight, have intensive rehabilitation in the physiotherapy department and delay a decision about surgery. Three years later Surgeon 'B' was being sued for procrastination because HD had now had a spinal fusion in another hospital with a good result. It was not sustained.

Surgeons must strike a fine balance between acknowledging the patient's freedom to choose, and recommending what they believe is in the patient's best interest. It is probably better to err on the side of not operating if the opinions of the surgeon and patient differ.

Surgeon's choice not to treat

Patients can sometimes be very manipulative and try to persuade surgeons to operate against their best judgement. However, doctors are free to accept or refuse to treat a patient. There are times when it is preferable that the surgeon refuses to treat. This depends of course on their professional obligations in an emergency or in an isolated community. Occasionally it is in the best interest of a difficult or aggressive patient that they be referred to another surgeon.

In spite of offering one's best advice, patients will sometimes seek a second opinion. This referral depends on agreement between the patient and doctor. Even though it suggests some lack of confidence, it is preferable to carrying out (or not carrying out) procedures that are thought to be inadvisable. It must be handled sensitively and should, if possible, be anticipated by suggesting a choice of appropriate colleagues.

REFERENCES

1. From dependence to partnership: patients redefine their role in health care (Editorial) *The Patient's Network* 1996; 1:1–7.
2. Richards T. Partnership with patients *BMJ* 1998; 316: 85–86.
3. Entwistle VA, Sheldon TA, Sowden AJ, *et al*. Supporting consumer involvement in decision making: what constitutes quality in consumer health information? *Int. J. Qual. Healthcare* 1996; 8: 425–437.
4. Meryn S. Improving doctor patient communication *BMJ* 1998; 316: 1922.
5. Makoul G, Arntson P, Schofield T. Health promotion in primary care: physician–patient communication and decision making about prescription medications *Soc. Sci. Med.* 1995; 41: 1241–1244.
6. See case of *Bolam* v. *Friern Hospital Management Committee* [1957] 2 All ER 118.
7. *Sidway* v. *Board of Governors of the Bethlem Royal Hospital and the Maudsley* [1985] AC 871, 1 All ER 643.
8. Godlee F. Applying research evidence to individual patients *BMJ* 1998; 316: 1621–1622.
9. *Rogers* v. *Whittaker* [1992] 67 AWR 47.
10. BMJ Legal Correspondent. What should the doctor tell? *BMJ* 1985; 290: 780–781.
11. Re W (a minor) (medical treatment) 1992; 4 All ER 627.
12. Lord Donaldson, MR, in *Re J* (a minor) (medical treatment) [1992] 4 All ER 614.
13. Mulcahy D, Cunningham K, McCormack D, *et al*. Informed consent from whom? *J. R. Coll. Surg. Edinburgh* 1997; 42. 161–164.
14. Richardson N, Jones P, Thomas M. Should house officers obtain consent for operations and anaesthesia? *Health Trends* 1996; 28: 56–58.

Chapter
4

POSITIONING OF THE PATIENT

The surgeon and the anaesthetist share the responsibility of caring for the patient whilst under the anaesthetic. There are particular risks related to the position of the patient which should be anticipated and avoided. Surgery to the lumbar spine is carried out with the patient in one of several positions.

1. Prone with the patient lying over a frame. The pelvis and the lower chest are supported by the periphery of the frame, which takes the weight of the trunk (*Figure 4.1*). The abdomen lies pendulous within the frame and it is free from pressure. This avoids compression of the inferior vena cava, and ensures that there is an unimpeded return of venous blood from the lower limbs to the heart. If there is pressure on the abdomen, venous blood tends to return to the heart partly via the plexus of veins within the spine – through Batson's extra dural venous plexus – and the surgeon can then expect copious

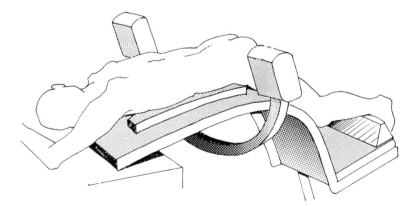

Figure 4.1. Diagram to show a patient lying on a spinal frame. The abdomen is pendulous through a hole in the frame. The 'U' arm of an image intensifier X-ray can be positioned across the table to identify the correct spinal levels for surgery.

bleeding from the spine. It therefore pays to make sure that the abdomen is free from any external pressure.

It is also important to be sure that there is not undue pressure from the frame on the groins, which might occlude the venous return from the lower limbs (see below).

2. Prone with the patient in the knee–elbow position. The patient kneels on the table. The abdomen is free from pressure and there is therefore even less intraspinal venous bleeding than would be expected lying on a frame. However, the hips are more flexed than when on a frame, and because of pressure in the groins in this position, it is associated with the occasional complications of hypotension, deep venous thrombosis and ischaemic muscle compartment syndrome [1, 2]. The undesirable effects are limited by preventing acute flexion of the lower limbs.

3. Lying on the side. If the patient lies on the side, the posterior spine can be approached whilst the surgeon is seated. There is no pressure on the abdomen. It has the advantage that the wound is kept relatively dry, as blood flows out of the wound from the operation site.

4. Supine. The patient is supine when the lumbar spine is approached anteriorly.

COMPLICATIONS

Deep venous thrombosis

Thrombosis of the deep veins will occur sub-clinically in many patients having spine surgery. However, clinical features of thrombosis – a painful tender calf, positive Holman's sign and slight pyrexia – occur in only about 3–4%. These patients require anticoagulant therapy to reduce the risk of pulmonary embolus. The risk of thrombosis is increased if a patient is in the knee–elbow position with a pillow tightly under the flexed knees, and if there is any pressure on the groins.

Post-operative hypotension

The perfusion of the lower limbs can be impaired during surgery in the knee–elbow position, with post-operative hyperaemia of the entire lower extremities. Post-operative hypotension may be due to the release of a tourniquet effect similar to the 'declamping phenomenon' seen after aorto-iliac occlusion. Most patients who have been in the knee–elbow position will have a short period of post-operative hypotension, and occasionally the degree and extent of the hypotension will cause concern. The risk is affected by the anaesthetic technique, obesity, the operation time, the extent of the surgical bleeding and particularly the degree of hip flexion.

Compartment syndrome

Patients in the knee–elbow position with the hips flexed can develop marked congestion and cyanosis of the lower limbs, especially if the patient is obese. It may occur from groin pressure when lying on a frame. If this is not noted on the operating table, and the circulation is not improved by either extending the lower limbs or relieving the groin pressure, these patients can develop bilateral calf muscle ischaemia and sometimes fatal renal failure. If muscle ischaemia is subsequently suspected, and confirmed by measuring compartment pressures, the muscle compartments should be surgically decompressed.

Peripheral nerve injury

Faulty positioning can cause peripheral nerve injuries if these nerves are subjected to pressure. This is prevented if both the surgeon and anaesthetist spend a few minutes at the start of the operation inspecting the patient's position, and making sure there is no localized pressure over areas at neurological risk.

The ulnar nerve is the most frequently reported peripheral nerve to be injured by malpositioning during surgery [3]. The arms and elbows are therefore positioned to avoid pressure on the ulnar nerves at the medial epicondyle. Soft padding may be required to redistribute the weight of the limb. Other nerves in the upper limb, such as the radial nerve or the brachial plexus, may be affected if they suffer from high localized pressure. The arms are best abducted at 90° and supported by pillows under the chest and by arm-boards on either side. This avoids pressure in the axilla and in the upper arm.

In the lower limb the femoral nerve, peroneal nerve and the lateral femoral cutaneous nerve are at risk. These nerves are vulnerable to direct pressure because of their proximity to bone or to traction when they are stretched across a highly mobile joint. It is the surgeon's responsibility to check that these respective sites are free of pressure or tension.

> **Case Report 8:** *Femoral nerve compression.* A 60-year-old obese lady had a discectomy at L5/S1. When she recovered from the anaesthetic she noticed that she had a new pain in the front of the right thigh. She was found to have an absent knee reflex and in the weeks after the operation she noted that the right leg was weak and there was marked wasting of the quadriceps muscle. Electrical studies confirmed the clinical impression that she had a femoral nerve lesion. There was no suggestion of a spinal problem affecting the roots of the femoral nerve.
>
> The doctor asked by the plaintiff's solicitor to investigate this complication, concluded that there was probably some localized pressure on the right femoral nerve during the operation when she was lying prone on the spinal frame. Although the surgeon and the anaesthetist were at a loss to explain how this could have happened, a settlement was made out of court.

Pressure sores

Small areas of the patient's skin may be exposed to high pressures if the load is not evenly distributed over a wide region. An unconscious patient cannot move to relieve pressure on a localized area, and unless the pressure points are protected, this can result in post-operative pressure sores.

For example, the front of the shin just above the ankle may be exposed to high pressure as the foot hangs freely over the end of the operating table. The sharp edge of the table can cause a line of high pressure over the front of the ankle. Similarly the side of the knee may take an excessive load if, as the leg lies externally rotated, the outer knee is allowed to press on a hard surface. And the scrotum can occasionally be caught in tight materials resulting in post-operative pain. Patients most at risk of skin problems are the elderly, those with rheumatoid arthritis, diabetes and those having steroid therapy.

Burns

Diathermy burns are unusual because of appropriate insulation, but if a diathermy forceps or needle carelessly lies in contact with the patient's skin, and the surgeon's foot accidentally rests on the pedal, there will be a burn.

Too liberal application of antiseptic skin preparation can cause irritant fluid to run far beyond the operation site to areas hidden by the towels, such as to the groins or the face. The preparation should therefore be limited to the immediate operation site. A few patients are sensitive to iodine, and if liquid iodine remains in contact with their skin for a long time, they will develop an unpleasant rash, skin blisters and sometimes permanent scarring.

REFERENCES

1. Alexander JP. Problems associated with the use of the knee–chest position for operations on lumbar intervertebral discs *J. Bone Jt. Surg.* 1973; 55-B: 279–284.
2. Aschoff A, Steiner-Milz, Steiner H-H. Lower limb compartment syndrome following lumbar discectomy in the knee–chest position *Neurosurgery Rev.* 1990; 13: 155–159.
3. Miller RG, Camp PE. Post operative ulnar neuropathy *JAMA* 1979; 17: 284–293.

Chapter
5

NERVE ROOT DAMAGE

Many patients who have surgery to the spine are fearful that they will suffer neurological injury. They have heard disastrous stories from friends, and have read about these problems in the newspapers. Nerve damage can occur in any spinal operation, and although not common, surgeons have a duty to warn about this possibility. A single nerve root injury can be transient or permanent. The latter is very troublesome. Multiple root injury is disastrous. The best method of management is prevention.

PATHOLOGICAL MECHANISM

Nerve roots can be damaged during open discectomy, decompression for stenosis and instrumentation during spinal fusion, or during subcutaneous procedures. Root problems can occur at a later stage as a consequence of surgery. There are many different causes of injury, and it is not always easy in retrospect to determine the exact mechanism.

Root manipulation

A nerve root can be damaged when manipulation of the root affects its blood supply. The root is particularly vulnerable if the blood supply is already precarious prior to surgery. A large disc protrusion which compresses the nerve root will cause increased intraradicular venous pressure. This reduces the blood flow and impairs the arterial supply to the root. There will be nerve root oedema as extravascular fluid collects in the root, and nerve function is then impaired. This contributes to the leg symptoms of sciatic pain, weakness and reduced reflexes.

When the surgeon or the assistant retracts a nerve root that has been under this type of compression, there is a risk that further disturbance of the root circulation will cause critical damage. The magnitude and reversibility of any neural dysfunction due to operative retraction depends on the amount of force applied and its duration [1]. The less force and the shorter its application the more likely the tissues are to recover. The nerve roots are more tolerant to pressure than is the spinal cord.

In one patient the root may be robust enough to withstand a degree of manipulation when the disc is being removed, and no damage will occur. However, in another, the root may be just functioning on a very limited blood supply, and slight manipulation during surgery can cause a critical problem. It is not possible for the surgeon to predict this complication. The disc is satisfactorily removed, but the patient wakes up from the anaesthetic to find that the nerve has been damaged. The pain is worse than before surgery and the leg is weak.

The nerve root usually lies directly over a protruding disc and it has to be retracted in order to remove the protrusion (*Figure 5.1*). The surgeon gently displaces the nerve root from the apex of the bulging disc so that the outer annulus of the disc can be incised and the protruding fragment extracted. Sometimes the fragment of disc has already extruded through the outer annulus, and it is directly pressing on the nerve root. The root still has to be moved to one side in order to remove the fragment. Whilst the surgeon extracts the disc fragment, the assistant has to hold the nerve root out of the way with a retractor.

It is during this period of displacing the root, and then holding it to one side with a retractor, that damage can occur. If the blood supply is already precarious, then manipulation of the root can further impair the circulation in that root and this may result in further damage.

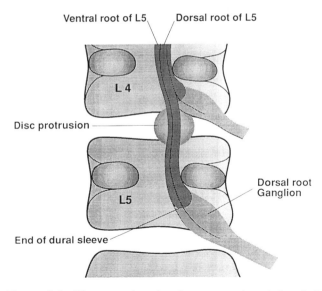

Figure 5.1. Diagram showing how a postero-lateral disc protrusion at L4/5 compresses the L5 root. The root has to be gently retracted, usually to the medial side in order to remove the protruding disc.

It is standard practice to handle nerve roots with great care, and to displace and retract them gently. The assistant is asked to release the traction on the nerve root every few minutes, in order that the blood supply will be periodically re-established. However, even when adopting this safe practice, from time to time nerve root damage will occur in expert hands. In addition, it is not possible to identify those patients at particular risk of this complication prior to surgery. It is only recognized when the patient recovers from the anaesthetic.

Root contusion

The nerve root may be damaged by contusion from a surgical instrument. It is called the 'battered root syndrome' [2]. The risk of intra-operative neural injury begins at the time of the sub-periosteal exposure of the posterior elements of the spine, when care should be taken to avoid inadvertent canal penetration. The risk is diminished if there has been careful pre-operative inspection of the radiographs to identify any mid-line spina bifida. A careful sub-periosteal dissection with a large elevator reduces the risk of penetrating a neural arch defect. If this should occur there will be an immediate pool of clear CSF indicating a dural tear. One then fears that there may have been associated root contusion.

It is essential to see both the root and the protruding disc. In order to obtain a satisfactory field of view, some of the inferior bony lamina of the vertebra above is often removed – a 'fenestration'. It is usually possible to see the L5/S1 disc without removing any of the bony lamina of L5, because the L5/S1 disc is immediately behind the inter-lamina space at L5/S1. Removing the ligamentum flavum between these two laminae provides sufficient space to see the nerve roots and the underlying disc. However, at L4/5 the disc is behind the lower aspect of the lamina of L4, and a fenestration of L4 lamina is required. Similarly a fenestration of L3 is necessary to expose the L3/4 disc.

In the process of performing a fenestration and nibbling away the lower margin of the lamina, a nerve root can be contused by the jaws of the nibbler. This is a particular risk if the spinal canal is narrow, causing the roots to be compressed tightly against the lamina. If the contusion is towards the mid-line, then the sacral roots are at risk, whilst if the contusion is lateral, one of the exiting lumbar roots is more likely to be involved.

The surgeon will be aware of possible damage to the mid-line sacral roots because there will be a leakage of cerebro-spinal fluid. The mid-line sacral roots are intradural in the lumbar spine and in order to contuse an intradural root, the dura is usually torn. At the lateral side of the canal, the nerve roots are partly extradural, and contusion can occur without a leak of cerebro-spinal fluid. The surgeon may be unaware of this nerve injury.

A nerve root can be damaged by an osteotome when decompressing a small spinal canal. Such a canal is constitutionally narrow and, with the addition of degenerative change, bone may be pressing on a nerve root. In the process of trimming the overhanging bone a nerve root may be contused. It is not always possible to see the root. It is then identified by 'feel'. It is protected by inserting a blunt instrument between the root and the bone. The root may be contused by the osteotome if its position is misjudged.

Diathermy

Electrocauterization of bleeding extradural veins may cause heat damage if a nerve root lies in close proximity to the electrode. A jerk of the leg warns the surgeon too late that this injury has occurred. Diathermy must therefore be used with great care in the extradural space, and then only when the nerve roots are under direct vision.

Root avulsion

Occasionally a nerve root may be avulsed if it is mistaken for disc material. It has been reported in 0.4% of patients having laminectomy [3]. The root can be stretched to a very thin ribbon over a protruding disc, and the surgeon may then mistake the root for the outer annulus of the disc. The dural sac is displaced medially, and by mistake an incision may be made in the very thin nerve root instead of in the annulus. A disc extractor is used to remove what is thought to be disc material, and a nerve root withdrawn instead. There is no alternative but to remove that section of the root, and accept that an unfortunate injury has occurred.

Nerve root damage is more common when there are conjoined nerve roots, which occur in about 5% of patients (*Figure 5.2*). The surgeon may visualize and protect what is believed to be the only root which is leaving the spine at that level, and be unaware that there is also an adjacent secondary root. If this is not seen, and it is unprotected, the conjoined root can be damaged. These adventitious roots can usually be recognized on the MRI scan (*Figure 5.3*), forewarning the surgeon of an increased risk of root injury.

Damage from instrumentation

When root damage occurs during spinal fusion, it is usually the result of contusion from the instrumentation. Sublaminar wires are sometimes used to apply and hold metalwork tightly to the lamina. As these wires are inserted, they can tear the dura and sometimes damage the underlying roots [4]. Patients with spinal stenosis are particularly at risk [5]. The surgeon cautiously identifies a site to position the wire by probing under the lamina with a blunt instrument. In a stenotic canal this can be difficult, and either the dura can be torn with damage to underlying roots or, more seriously, a wire may be passed under a root, guillotining the root as the wire is tightened. The surgeon may be unaware of damage until the patient awakens from the anaesthetic.

Pedicle screws are the most common method of spinal fixation at the present time. The surgeon identifies the anatomical site to introduce the screw. This is on the lateral aspect of the lamina at the intersection of two lines, one

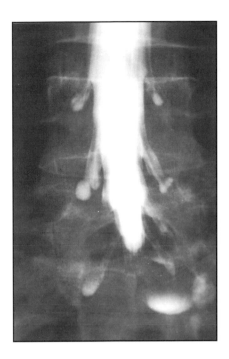

Figure 5.2. Radiculogram showing conjoint roots (with asymptomatic arachnoid sacculations at the end of the dural sleeves).

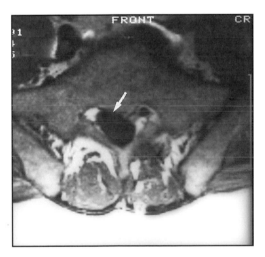

Figure 5.3. Conjoined roots which are iso-intense with the dural sac.

vertically through the mid-line of the facet joint, and the other transversely along the transverse process.

The perpendicular track down the pedicle is developed first by drilling usually with a 3.5 mm bit, and then tapping. A blunt probe ensures that the peripheral cortex of the pedicle has not been transgressed. The site for the placement of the screw is identified into the vertebral body, its length determined by a depth gauge, and a screw is then introduced.

Each lumbar and sacral vertebra has a slightly different anatomy, and there is also individual variation. Placement of sacral screws can be difficult. The thoracic spine can present problems, when an open-lamina technique reduces the risk of inaccurate placement [6]. It is not surprising, therefore, that even in expert hands the pedicle is transgressed and the peripheral cortex broken in about 12–21% of screw placements [7, 8]. A pre-operative CT helps accurate placement.

Screws that do not perforate more than 4 mm do not usually cause neurological problems. This is because there is usually ample space between the pedicle and nerve root. Occasionally, however, a screw or a splinter of bone can damage a nerve root running close to the medial side or the undersurface of the pedicle. The degree of damage depends on whether the root is irritated, contused or transfixed. If the screw is placed too medially the dura may be penetrated, or if the screw goes too deep visceral damage can occur.

Percutaneous damage

Nerve roots are at risk during percutaneous procedures. They are liable to injury when needles, cannulae and probes are introduced into the spine for diagnosis and therapy. These procedures include diagnostic probing, nerve root injections, discograms, facet joint injections, chymopapain, endoscopic discectomy, laser treatment.

Percutaneous procedures are therefore normally carried out with enough sedation to make the procedure tolerable, but not too much to prevent co-operation. There is interaction between the surgeon and patient so that if the instrument approaches a nerve root, the patient can immediately give warning, and the instrument is then replaced. Touching a root with a needle does no harm, but transfixing a root or injecting toxic substances can cause structural damage. There is probably a minority of responsible surgeons who would carry out theraputic percutaneous procedures under general anaesthetic, but most surgeons would think that this is not best practice because of the risk of nerve root damage.

Fat graft

The development of fibrosis after decompressive surgery may be responsible for stenotic symptoms at a later stage. Some surgeons prefer to apply a fat graft over the dura at the site of decompression to minimize this scarring. The fat is loosely laid over the dura in the hope that it will prevent a layer of fibrosis forming as a post-laminectomy membrane. Unfortunately the fat can migrate into the proximal spinal canal and compress the cauda equina causing multiple root compression or even a post-operative cauda equina syndrome. Once recognized it needs urgent decompression.

Multiple root damage

Multiple root injury after lumbar spine surgery is uncommon and it suggests rough handling of the tissues. There may be excessive and/or lengthy medial traction on the dural sac in order to expose a lateral disc protrusion. Several roots can then be devascularized, and fail to regain their normal function.

The roots may be devitalized from the pressure of packing when trying to prevent bleeding. Applying packs is, of course, legitimate in order to see the operation site, but if packing is excessive, it can affect the blood supply to the nerves which may not recover.

Post-operative root pathology

In the early post-operative period root symptoms may recur as a result of a new disc protrusion, when a further fragment extrudes to compress the nerve root. The same root symptoms may be the result of a post-operative haematoma.

A dural tear during surgery may cause a pseudomeningocele post-operatively. Its incidence after lumbar spine surgery has been estimated at between 0.07 and 2% [9]. This false sac may subsequently entrap with a ball valve effect, one or more nerve roots causing pain and dysfunction. This complication should be considered in any patient who slowly develops multiple root problems after surgery. It can occur weeks or years after surgery (see Chapter 6).

If, some months after surgery, the two vertebrae settle together following a rather radical discectomy or because of post-operative discitis, root pain can occur when the nerve root becomes entrapped in the root canal.

POST-OPERATIVE SYMPTOMS AND SIGNS

When a nerve root has been damaged during surgery, as the patient recovers from the anaesthetic they are immediately aware of sensory and motor symptoms. If, however, there is a recurrent disc protrusion or a haematoma there may be a period of reasonable comfort followed in a few hours by the development of new root symptoms. It is not always easy to distinguish these various causes of post-operative root pain from clinical assessment.

The sensory symptoms may be numbness or pain.

- If a nerve has been contused, or its blood supply damaged by retraction, the patient usually has severe post-operative pain in the root distribution. They also have sensory loss.
- By contrast, when a nerve has been divided or avulsed, the patient is aware of loss of sensation in the nerve root distribution, but does not usually have pain.
- Whatever the pathology, the anaesthesia is in the distribution of the nerve root. The L5 root generally supplies the calf and the big toe, whilst the S1 root supplies the outer calf and the outer foot. However, because there is

considerable variation between the root distribution, the sensory change will vary from one patient to another. Vague generalized leg pain is not usually root pain.

- Patients with a recurrent disc or with a haematoma have both pain and numbness.

The motor component of the root damage causes,

- weakness of the muscles supplied by the nerve, and again this varies between patients. An S1 root injury may cause complete foot drop in one patient and no noticeable weakness in another,
- most muscles and most areas of the skin are supplied by two nerve roots, and therefore if there is no pain, a single root injury may be tolerated reasonably well.

Multiple root damage to the S2–4 nerve roots can be disastrous because these nerves supply the bladder, the bowel and the sexual organs.

- A single sacral root lesion can be well tolerated, but injury to more than one sacral root is a major problem.
- The degree of disfunction can vary between patients.
- Impairment of the sensory component will affect the bladder, bowel and sexual sensation, and injury to the motor nerves will disturb micturition, bowel evacuation and ejaculation.
- The same nerves supply the anal skin and muscles and damage will result in peri-anal anaesthesia and loss of anal muscle tone.

MANAGEMENT

If a patient complains of severe pain in a root distribution after surgery, and perhaps numbness and weakness, the surgeon has to think about the possibility of a lesion that requires urgent repeat surgery.

Surgical damage

When the surgeon is aware that nerve root damage occurred at the time of surgery, there is generally little that can be done to rectify the situation. The patient may complain of severe root pain, numbness and weakness when they recover from the anaesthetic, but the damage has been done to the nerve root by retraction or contusion. Alternatively, if there is not pain but only numbness and weakness, this suggests that a nerve root has been divided or avulsed, and again a re-operation is not likely to help. The damage has been done. It is not correctable and it is too late. These patients need long-term assistance by Pain Specialists to help with their disability.

However, the operation may have been uneventful, and immediate post-operative symptoms of severe pain may indicate that there is an obviously treatable cause. The root may be irritated or compressed by pedicle screw and early corrective surgery can be effective. Imaging is usually inappropriate, because of the scattering effect of metal. Damage from instrumentation can be assumed and it needs to be repositioned or removed by early surgery.

A new post-operative lesion

There may be a new lesion that develops in the post-operative hours which can and should be effectively treated. This may cause the same symptoms of root pain, numbness and weakness because there is

- a new fragment of disc material which has extruded and is compressing the root
- a gathering haematoma.

The temporal sequence

The timing when the symptoms occur is helpful when making the diagnosis about these treatable conditions. If, after a baseline of a normal neurological examination, there develops progressive root pain, numbness and weakness in the 48 hours after surgery, this suggests a new lesion – a disc fragment or haematoma. If, on the other hand, the symptoms are marked and they do not change from the time the patient recovered from the anaesthetic, this is suggestive of root damage at the time of surgery. Unfortunately, the symptoms may appear to deteriorate only because the patient is becoming more aware of the problem as they slowly regain consciousness and as they have less sedation. In reality the pathology may not have changed.

Any patient therefore who complains of post-operative root pain and who had troublesome numbness and weakness which is more severe than the pre-operative symptoms, requires urgent assessment by the surgeon. The neurological state needs to be carefully assessed and recorded, and the wound inspected. Urgent MRI imaging is considered if there might be a new disc herniation or haematoma.

MRI will help diagnose a recurrent disc herniation. Although the imaging is not always conclusive, there is usually marked displacement of the thecal sac. Gadolinium-enhanced MRI is more helpful some weeks after the first operation than in the earlier period (see below).

A haematoma will be suspected from bleeding or swelling of the wound. The MRI will show its presence and extent (*Figure 5.4*), and it requires urgent evacuation to decompress the nerve root.

Careful post-operative assessment is essential, because a progressive lesion is usually reversible if it is recognized and treated promptly. It is better to err on the side of re-operation if there is a possibility that the root problem is treatable. There is a possibility of recovery if a further disc fragment is removed, or if a haematoma is evacuated.

Late post-operative lesion

MRI is an important investigation for every patient with post-operative root symptoms when there are new abnormal neurological signs. It may show a

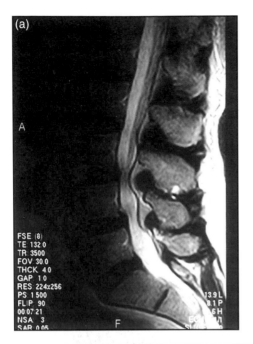

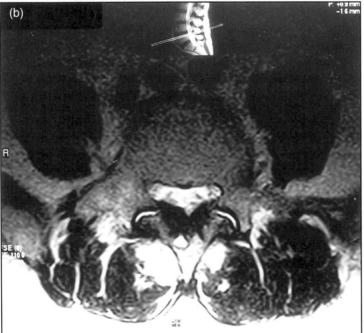

Figure 5.4(a). MRI showing post-operative compression of the dural sac at L3/4 and L4/5 with the dura displaced anteriorly some way up the lumbar canal. Transverse image **(b)** shows this displacement is compatible with a haematoma.

pseudo-meningocele with root entrapment or some other unsuspected pathology like a new disc protrusion, low grade discitis or a previously unsuspected tumour.

Scar formation is an inevitable consequence of surgery, and it probably does not cause symptoms. New disc material, however, may be symptomatic. It is not easy to distinguish normal scar from a new fragment of disc material. Gadolinium, when injected intravenously, will deposit in aqueous solutions if there is a blood supply, and it brightens the water protons on MRI–T1 weighted images. It therefore has the capacity to distinguish between scar and a recurrent disc fragment (*Figures 5.5* and *5.6*).

Post-operative cauda equina syndrome (see Chapter 6)

Multiple sacral root damage will cause numbness in the perineum, scrotum and peri-anal region. Any patient who says that they have numbness in this

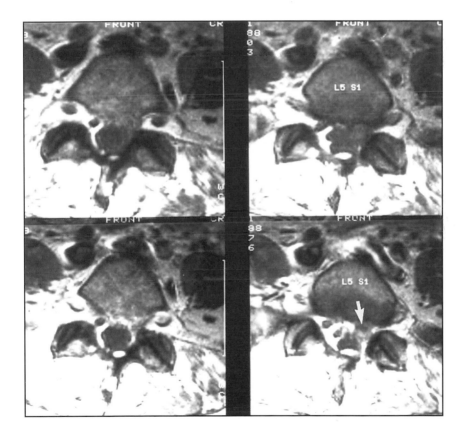

Figure 5.5. MRI of a patient with recurrent disc symptoms after surgery. The top two images are without gadolinium. The bottom two are with gadolinium and on the right there are non-enhancing echoes compatible with a recurrent fragment of disc.

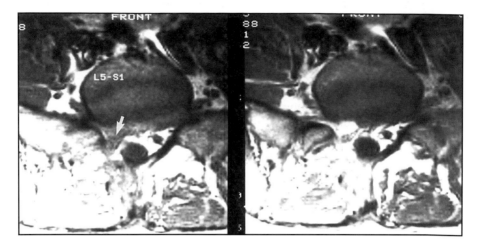

Figure 5.6. MRI of a patient with recurrent disc symptoms after surgery. The image on the left without gadolinium (arrow) could be scar tissue or a disc fragment. On the right with gadolinium it uniformly enhances and is obviously scar.

distribution needs urgent and careful neurological assessment. Sacral root damage also causes loss of anal muscle tone and bladder problems. There may be loss of urinary sensation, or an inability to pass urine, but it is difficult to detect this in a nervous patient in the early post-operative period.

It is the distribution of sensory loss and the reduced anal muscle tone that is important diagnostically. These patients need urgent imaging with MRI and re-operation to remove any treatable compressing lesion. The sooner the roots are decompressed, the more likely the patient is to recover. Delay can be costly. It is better to re-explore the wound without MRI if this is not readily available.

The sacral roots are especially sensitive to compression, and they may not recover even with rapid decompression.

PROGNOSIS

This is variable. It depends on the root(s) involved, the cause and the extent of the damage and personal variations in the neurological anatomy.

A root which has been divided or avulsed will not recover. Patients will generally come to terms with the numbness. Initially it is annoying and is a nuisance, but patients gradually forget the loss of sensation unless they are reminded of it. Most of the skin is supplied by two nerve roots, and this overlap means that with loss of one root, the skin sensation, although generally reduced, is not totally absent. However, weakness because of paralysed muscle is a considerable disability. It is less easily accepted, especially if there is a foot drop. Minor weakness may be treated with an orthosis, and more marked weakness with foot surgery.

A contused root, or a root damaged by retraction is initially very painful, and it recovers only partially and slowly. Many patients continue with severe disabling pain for many years. They complain that the pain is stabbing, shooting, burning and very unpleasant. Pain can not be measured objectively, and one has to take at face value the patient's complaints. However, contused nerves at other sites tend to become less painful with time and, although the nerve sensation may never fully recover, a degree of improvement can be expected.

Roots which are compressed by fragments of disc or by haematoma and which are not treated surgically, tend to become less painful with time, but the numbness and weakness usually remain.

The chances of recovery from multiple sacral root injury is poor. Partially compressed roots causing patchy numbness are more likely to recover than roots which have complete loss of function. However, when neurological damage is more complete, affecting the bladder, bowel and sexual function, it does not usually recover. Patients have to learn the technique of self-catheterization and daily manual evacuation of the bowels. Their life expectancy is reduced because repeated urinary tract infections will damage the kidney.

Nerve root injury is best prevented because recovery is poor and definitive treatment does not usually exist. The risk is reduced by careful pre-operative planning, by an awareness of the dangers, meticulous haemostasis, adequate lighting and a careful operative technique.

Case Report 9: *Laser discectomy.* Mr MJ was 32 years of age and had a 7-month history of back pain and right sciatica into the calf. SLR was 50/80. He was having difficulty keeping at work and was advised by friends to have laser discectomy. He remembers being told that most people do well with this procedure, although occasionally there can be a flare, with symptoms getting worse in the first few days after treatment. If unsuccessful, surgery would be required to remove a disc fragment and/or decompress the spinal canal.

He was given a general anaesthetic and, when he recovered from the operation, he knew immediately that there was a new and more severe pain in the right leg down to the foot. He was told that this would probably settle down and was discharged home the following day.

Mr MJ continued with this severe right leg pain, and obtained a second opinion from a neurologist. He was told that a nerve root had probably been irritated by the percutaneous procedure and that it would probably settle with time. Unfortunately, he continued with unpleasant leg pain for more than 3 years after the laser treatment.

He sued the surgeon for not telling him of the risk, and for damaging the root. He believed that the procedure should have been carried out under sedation and not under general anaesthetic so that he could have warned the surgeon if the procedure was disturbing the nerve root.

The surgeon said that he always told patients of the risk of nerve root damage. The letter to the general practitioner prior to surgery said that risks and benefits were described, but root injury was not specified. It was successfully defended on the grounds that even if he had been told of possible root damage, it is probable that he would still have chosen to have the procedure. In addition, it was accepted that there is a small body of responsible practitioners who would have carried out this procedure under general anaesthetic.

> **Case Report 10:** *Too strong retraction.* Mr FL was a 48-year-old mechanic with a history of back pain and 4 months of severe left-sided sciatica. An MRI scan showed a large disc protrusion at L4/5, degenerate facet joints and some canal stenosis. During a discectomy the surgeon recorded that the dura was damaged, and that strong retraction of the nerve roots was necessary in order to remove the sequestrated disc. Post-operatively, Mr FL had numbness in the peri-anal region, and an inability to pass urine. This did not recover.

Mr FL claimed that the surgeon had not taken into account the respect that was required for the nerve roots. It was agreed that a single nerve root injury might occur even when exercising great care, but multiple nerve root damage associated with a dural tear and a description of strong retraction was not defensible.

REFERENCES

1. Dahlin LB, Rydevik B, McLean WG. Changes in fast axonal transport during experimental nerve compression at low pressures *Exp. Neurol.* 1984; 84: 29–34.
2. Bertrand G. The battered root problem *Orthop. Clin. N Am.* 1975; 6: 305–310.
3. Mayfield F. Complications of laminectomy *Clin. Neurosurg.* 1975; 23: 435–439.
4. Goll SR, Balderston RA, Stambough JL, *et al.* Depth of intraspinal wire penetration during the passage of sublaminar wires *Spine* 1988; 13: 503–509.
5. Dove J. Neurological deterioration after posterior wiring of the cervical spine *J. Bone Jt. Surg.* 1998; 80-B: 555.
6. Xu R, Ebraheim NA, Yianjia O. Anatomic considerations of pedicle screw placement in the thoracic spine *Spine* 1998; 23: 1065–1068.
7. Liljenqvist U, Halm H, Link T. Accuracy of pedicle screw placement in scoliosis surgery by means of computed tomography *J. Bone Jt. Surg.* 1998; 80-B: Suppl 1: 92.
8. Laine T, Makitalo K, Schlenzka D, Tallroth K, Poussa M, Alho A. Accuracy of pedicle screw insertion: a prospective CT study in 30 low back patients *Eur. Spine* 1987; 6: 402–405.
9. Hadani FG, Knoler N, Tadmor R *et al.* Entrapped lumbar nerve root in pseudomeningocele after laminectomy: report of three cases *Neurosurgery* 1986; 19: 405–407.

Chapter
6

CAUDA EQUINA SYNDROME

Cauda equina syndrome is the result of major compression of the whole or part of the cauda equina, causing impairment of the circulation of the nerve roots and failure of nerve function. This involves the sacral nerve roots but sometimes the lumbar roots also, depending on the level and the completeness of the lesion. The important clinical problem is loss of control of the bladder, bowels and sexual function. These are controlled by the sacral nerve roots.

ANATOMY

The cauda equina is a bundle of nerve roots within the lumbar and sacral spinal canal (*Figure 6.1*). The spinal cord ends at the lower border of L2. Below this, the lumbar and sacral nerve roots continue as the cauda equina (*Figure 6.2*). Each root is supplied by a radicular artery. This is a branch of a lumbar artery which arises from the aorta. The flow is centripetal, from the intervertebral foramen, the artery ascending proximally in the nerve root towards the conus.

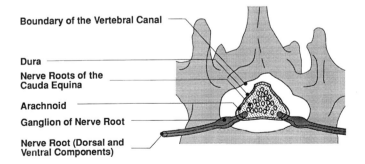

Boundary of the Vertebral Canal

Dura

Nerve Roots of the Cauda Equina

Arachnoid

Ganglion of Nerve Root

Nerve Root (Dorsal and Ventral Components)

Figure 6.1. Diagram to show the cross-section of the lumbar spine, with the cauda equina in the spinal canal.

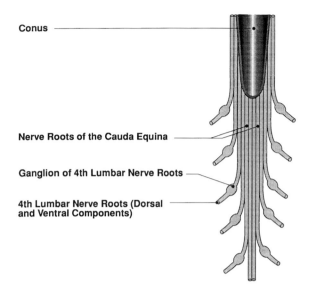

Conus

Nerve Roots of the Cauda Equina

Ganglion of 4th Lumbar Nerve Roots

4th Lumbar Nerve Roots (Dorsal and Ventral Components)

Figure 6.2. The conus is the lower end of the spinal cord. It terminates at L2, with the nerve roots continuing in the spinal canal as the cauda equina.

The flow can be reversed if there is pressure on the nerve root, because the vessels in the lower part of the spinal cord anastamose with the radicular vessels. The nerve roots are separate and are bathed in cerebro-spinal fluid within the dural membrane, and therefore there is no opportunity for a vascular anastomosis between the nerve roots. The sacral roots are posterior and in the mid-line of the cauda equina, and selective compression or injury at this site can have serious consequences.

PATHOLOGY

A low grade (partial) compression can be tolerated by the nerve roots. The arterial circulation may still provide an adequate supply of oxygen. However, a high pressure (complete) compression can devascularize the roots and this will permanently affect their function. There are several compressive lesions which can cause a cauda equina syndrome, such as a large disc protrusion, tumour, fracture, haemorrhage, abscess or iatrogenic injury.

Disc herniation

A lumbar disc herniation may at times occur so suddenly and be so massive that the whole of the cauda equina is seriously compressed. Generally a disc will protrude postero-laterally and it compresses only one, or perhaps two, nerve roots at the side of the cauda equina. It will cause sciatic pain down one leg in the distribution of the root(s). But on occasions, either as migration of a large fragment towards the mid-line, or as a herniation through the mid-line of the posterior annulus, the compression can be so severe as to involve all the cauda equina (*Figure 6.3*). It may be sudden or slowly progressive. The degree of compression will depend on the size of the herniated fragment, and the available space within the spinal canal. The roots within a small stenotic canal are particularly at risk from massive compression.

Spinal tumour

Tumours in the lumbar spine can compress the cauda equina, but unless there is bleeding into the tumour, the symptoms develop slowly. The diagnosis is often late, but it is usually made before the neurological lesion is complete.

Fracture

A fragment of bone from a burst fracture, which is displaced posteriorly, can damage the cauda equina, but it is surprising how often the nerve roots are spared even when there is a massive fragment in the spinal canal. In addition, displaced bone can remodel and fragments within the spinal canal can resorb, so the size of a fragment is not in itself an indication to operate. Conservative treatment is appropriate, unless the intraspinal bony fragment is causing neurological problems (see Chapter 14). However, some patients with a major wedge compression fracture and minimal neurological symptoms will get worse over the following months if the angular compression increases. This is more likely if the vertebra is wedged more than 30°.

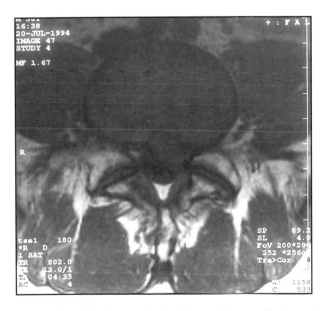

Figure 6.3. MRI of a patient with sudden partial cauda equina syndrome. There is a massive central and left-sided disc compressing the dural sac.

Haemorrhage

A post-operative haematoma needs to be excluded as a cause of unexpected neurological compression after surgery because, if unrelieved, it can steadily increase and cause a cauda equina syndrome. Sudden spontaneous extradural bleeding may occur in patients with bleeding diseases, and in traumatized patients whose spines are rigid from ankylosis spondylitis. This usually affects the spinal cord within the thoracic spine. There is more available extradural space in the lumbar spine, and the nerve roots are more forgiving than the spinal cord.

Infection

An abscess causing neurological compression in the lumbar region is rare. It is usually diagnosed early and effectively treated. In the thoracic spine, however, pyogenic and tuberculous abscesses can either compress the cord or occlude its blood supply with disastrous results.

Iatrogenic cauda equina syndrome

This is always very distressing. It can result from crushing the roots by instruments, compression from metalwork such as laminar hooks or wires, retraction whilst obtaining a good exposure, or a post-operative haematoma. Occasionally, fat graft applied to a decompressed area in the hope of preventing scarring, can migrate into the proximal spinal canal and compress the nerve roots.

Because the sacral roots are in the mid-line of the cauda equina, retraction from the lateral aspect must be heavy and prolonged to cause major problems. However, these roots are particularly vulnerable to crushing when the lamina is being removed in the mid-line, or when sublaminar wires are being threaded under the lamina. The surgeon exercises great caution at this site, especially if there is some spinal stenosis.

It is sometimes suggested that cauda equina syndrome can occur during an operation as a result of sudden unexpected loss of the blood supply to many nerve roots. This severe neurological complication can occur to the spinal cord in the thoracic and upper lumbar region, where one vessel will supply a large segment of the cord. Even gentle manipulative procedures can cause arterial spasm or thrombosis. This is serious at the level of the spinal cord, but in the lower lumbar region, where each nerve root of the cauda equina is supplied by its own artery, it is difficult to see how multiple roots can be similarly affected at the same time.

CLINICAL PRESENTATION

The term cauda equina syndrome is reserved for those patients who have severe bilateral sciatica, significant bilateral weakness, especially below the knees, saddle hypoaesthesia or anaesthesia and incontinence or retention of urine [1]. The frequency of this syndrome ranges from 1 to 10% of operated discs, depending on how rigorously the criteria are applied [2]. Ten percent of operated discs do not have bladder problems!

The onset of symptoms may be sudden, complete and dramatic. Alternatively, they can be slowly progressive, depending on the underlying pathology. The condition may progress to become complete or may remain incomplete. A careful on-going clinical assessment is essential, because once the diagnosis of cauda equina syndrome is made, delay in treatment can be disastrous.

A partial lesion is recognized by slowly developing bladder symptoms. The patient may admit to some difficulty passing urine, but can still manage to void voluntarily. They have partial sensory reduction around the anus, or a steadily increasing area of sensory loss. They tend to have unilateral symptoms, rather than pain equally in both legs. They may not develop faecal incontinence until a late stage.

Some patients with a symptomatic disc protrusion have difficulty passing urine, which is quite unrelated to any sacral nerve root problem. They simply have severe back pain which, in itself, can inhibit micturition. This is especially a problem when they are asked to pass urine whilst lying down. However, any patient with urinary difficulty needs a careful neurological assessment. If there are any signs of motor or sensory loss in a sacral root distribution, the bladder symptoms are then taken seriously.

URGENCY OF SURGERY

Traditional teaching is that this is an emergency. Once cauda equina syndrome is suspected, there needs to be urgent investigation with MRI or, if this is not available, CT or myelogram. It has been suggested that myelography might convert an incipient/incomplete/partial cauda equina syndrome into a complete lesion, and MRI is therefore the imaging of choice. If this confirms the diagnosis of a large compressive lesion, emergency surgery is required.

It is logical that the earlier the nerve roots are relieved of the compression and root circulation restored, the better will be the neurological recovery. However, there are reports in the literature that there is no relation between the timing of surgery and the degree of recovery. In fact, patients having later surgery seem to do better than those having earlier treatment. This anomaly defies logic, unless these reported series include patients with complete lesions who are treated by emergency surgery, and patients with incomplete lesions whose operation is delayed. Incomplete lesions have a propensity to recover, whilst patients with complete lesions generally reach the operating theatre in time for successful surgery. There is no responsible spinal surgeon who would delay operating on a cauda equina lesion because procrastination might give better results. However, it is not always easy for the litigant to argue that delay in surgery affected the eventual outcome.

Experimental work in animals has suggested that there is no difference in the extent of recovery whether the decompression is relieved immediately or at intervals of up to a week [3]. Work on monkeys has suggested that decompression within 1 hour of compression produces significant improvement, but this does not occur at 4 hours [4]. These studies probably relate to a complete lesion. If surgery can be carried out before retention of urine occurs, the prognosis is probably better [5, 6].

Patients with incomplete lesions have a good chance of recovering bladder function with decompressive surgery. Moller and Sogaard, who reviewed 63 patients who were decompressed after sustaining only partial cauda equina lesions, noted that in 97% the symptoms were relieved completely [7]. In 27 of these patients, the time from first symptoms to surgery was more than 24 hours.

An iatrogenic cauda equina syndrome requires similar urgent management. A recurrence of protrusion, haematoma, fat graft migration all deserve prompt intervention. Compressive sublaminar wires or hooks should be removed. However, there is no remedy for roots traumatized by instruments or by heavy retraction.

RECOVERY OF NERVE FUNCTION

Incomplete lesions

There is a capacity for some recovery in partial lesions if the compression is removed. Without surgery the prognosis is poor – bladder and bowel function tend not to improve and the lesion may progress to become complete. However, there is anecdotal evidence that an occasional patient who refuses surgery can make quite a good recovery. This is probably because a partial lesion from disc protrusion can recover to some extent as the inflammatory process resolves. It would not be grounds for operative delay. A significant degree of saddle anaesthesia carries a poor prognosis for recovery of bladder and bowel function [1].

Complete lesions

Depending on the severity and the duration of the compression, the chance of recovery is small. If there is absolute loss of oxygenation to nerve tissue for more than a few minutes, recovery is improbable. Thus, patients who have a sudden onset of major cauda equina symptoms are unlikely to improve with emergency surgery. Irreversible damage has already been done. However, there will be a few patients with sudden symptoms who clinically seem to have a major complete lesion but the loss of arterial supply is not absolute. Presumably these are the few patients with clinically complete lesions who do improve with early surgery. One therefore cannot presume that a cauda equina syndrome is irreversible, and all spinal surgeons would advise decompression as early as possible, even though the prognosis is poor for the complete lesion.

Case Report 11: *A sudden catastrophe.* Mr CJ was a 28-year-old factory worker. He had had low back pain and left sciatica for 6 weeks and his doctor had requested a hospital outpatient appointment. However, whilst waiting for this appointment, he was in his greenhouse at 12:00 h when he suddenly felt both his legs go numb. He had to crawl back into the house. He took two analgesics and went to bed. When he awoke 2 hours later his legs were still numb. His wife called the general practitioner and he was sent to hospital arriving at 17:00 h. The house officer noted numbness at the back of both legs, saddle anaesthesia and loss of anal tone. He had not passed urine for several hours. He was admitted and was catheterized.

The registrar saw him at 18:00 h and he advised that he should be observed overnight. The consultant did not know of his admission until the next day, and he then arranged for urgent transfer to a neurosurgical unit. An MRI scan showed a massive disc at L4/5 and this was removed at 16:00 h – 28 hours after the onset.

There was a negligence claim that the doctors had failed to recognize the urgency of the cauda equina syndrome, and consequently there was delay in decompression which gave a poor result. The defence argued successfully that, as a result of the sudden onset of the lesion and its complete nature, it was probable that surgery after 6 hours of the onset of symptoms would not have resulted in any recovery. Failure to recognize the urgency of the situation was not acceptable but it was agreed that it would probably not have affected the outcome.

REFERENCES

1. Kostuik JP. Current Opinion *Orthopaedics* 1993, 4: 11, 125.
2. Shapiro S. Cauda equina syndrome secondary to lumbar disc herniation *Neurosurgery* 1993, 32: 743–747.
3. Delamarter RB, Sherman JE, Carr JB. Cauda equina syndrome: neurologic recovery following immediate, early, or late decompression *Spine* 1991, 16: 1022–1029.
4. Stephenson GC. Acute cauda equina compression in a primate model. Evaluation or early surgery. MD Thesis, University of Leeds 1991.
5. Fager CA. Ruptured median and paramedian lumbar disc. A review of 243 cases *Surg. Neurol.* 1985, 23: 309–323.
6. Gleave JR, Macfarlane R. Prognosis for recovery of bladder function following lumbar central disc prolapse *B. J. Neurosurg.* 1990, 4: 205–209.
7. Moller CM, Sogaard I. The partial cauda equina syndrome *Ugeskr Laeg.* 1995; 157: 4567–4563.

Chapter

7

DAMAGE TO THE DURA

The dural membrane surrounding the cauda equina is sometimes damaged during lumbar spine surgery. It is not a major problem if it is carefully managed.

ANATOMY

There are really two layers of closely applied membrane surrounding the cauda equina. The outer membrane is the thicker dura and within it is the more delicate arachnoid (see *Figure 6.1*). If both are cut or torn, it is immediately obvious because there is a leak of clear cerebro-spinal fluid into the wound. If the dura alone is incised there will be no leak of cerebro-spinal fluid, but the arachnoid will bulge through the gaping dura.

METHOD OF INJURY

A dural tear occurs in about 3–5% of lumbar spine operations [1]. Patients having repeat surgery are at greater risk.

- It can occur in patients with spina-bifida occulta. In these patients, instead of the neural arch being complete posteriorly, there is a defect in the bone which is filled with fibrous tissue. During operative exposure to clear the laminae of soft tissue, a blunt instrument can penetrate through the laminar defect. This is avoidable if the surgeon studies the pre-operative X-ray and recognizes the presence of the spina-bifida occulta;
- the dura can be incised accidentally when gaining access to the spinal canal through the ligamentum flavum. The surgeon should incise the ligamentum flavum cautiously and slowly, stopping as soon as the underlying dura is visible. Magnification with enhanced lighting is helpful. After the first incision, the ligament is lifted up with a small hook or with dissectors whilst a piece is excised to gain access to the spinal canal. The dura is closely applied to the back of the ligament, especially if there is large disc

protrusion or spinal stenosis, and it can occasionally be cut, even when taking great care. It is better practice to excise a piece of ligamentum flavum, rather than tearing or ripping it with rongeurs. If both the dura and arachnoid are cut, there will be an obvious leak of cerebro-spinal fluid;

- the dura can also be torn when retracting the theca or when using blunt dissection to free an adherent nerve root from a disc protrusion;
- the dura can be nipped in the jaws of a bone rongeur if the foot-plate is not perpendicular to the bone that is to be removed;
- if the lamina is being removed with a bone drill, slippage of the drill can damage the dura. When decompressing a stenotic spine with thick laminae, dural damage is reduced if the lamina is first thinned with a drill before using rongeurs. The dura is also less likely to be damaged if, when using a drill, the surgeon works from the medial to the lateral side of the lamina;
- when repeating surgery, the scarred dura can easily be damaged by a tear or by an incision. It is wise to begin the dissection in virgin territory and work towards the area where the dura is scarred and vulnerable. It is technically difficult to work from medial to lateral side, and safer to begin at the lateral aspect of the dural sac.

IMMEDIATE CONSEQUENCES OF DURAL INJURY

All spine surgeons will occasionally damage the dura, and it must be accepted as a risk, even in expert hands. Unfortunately, once cerebro-spinal fluid is leaking into the wound, the operation becomes more difficult. The field of vision is impaired, not only because of the intermittent flow of clear fluid into the wound, but also because of venous bleeding. Although in many spinal operations it is difficult to avoid some bleeding from the extradural veins, the pressure of the intact dural sac generally keeps these veins compressed, and bleeding is usually minimal. When leaking cerebro-spinal fluid releases this pressure, the veins become congested and they can bleed copiously.

SURGICAL MANAGEMENT

When the dura is cut but the arachnoid remains intact, the dural tear will expand and the arachnoid and possibly nerve roots will bulge through the defect. The dura therefore needs to be repaired.

When both dura and arachnoid are cut, there is leaking cerebro-spinal fluid. Views differ about the best management. Many surgeons believe that a torn or cut dura should be repaired with fine sutures. Dorsal tears are easier to repair than those in a lateral position. Perhaps a small cut is best treated that way, with a small 6.0 suture. It is acceptable, however, to leave a dural tear unrepaired, placing blood clot, muscle patch or Gelfoam over the area as a seal. A larger tear can be repaired with a continuous suture without applying tension to the opposed edges. If it is decided not to repair the dura, because leaking cerebro-spinal fluid will affect the field of vision, a patty (a small soft swab) is placed over the defect as a temporary seal for the duration of the operation.

When the dura has been repaired, some surgeons will use the Queckenstedt test to increase the cerebro-spinal fluid pressure, and confirm that the closure is secure.

It is essential that there is a good tight fascial repair at the end of the operation, otherwise a post-operative leak of cerebro-spinal fluid can fill a dead space and become the site for a pseudomeningocele. Some surgeons prefer not to use a wound drain, whilst others believe that intermittent drainage is helpful.

LATE CONSEQUENCES OF A DURAL TEAR

A reduction in the volume of cerebro-spinal fluid will cause post-operative headache. This may last for a few days and it helps to nurse the patient flat for 2 days. The wound should be inspected daily to make sure that there is no leak of cerebro-spinal fluid into the dressings. Leakage usually stops if the patient remains flat. It is when the flow ceases, however, that there is a risk of meningitis from ascending infection, and therefore prophylactic antibiotics are necessary. If a cerebro-spinal fluid leak persists for more than 10 days, surgical repair should be considered.

A pseudomeningocele

A pseudomeningocele should be considered in a patient who has

- headache when assuming the erect posture
- a wound swelling

even if the surgeon was not aware of dural damage at the time of surgery.

A false sac of cerebro-spinal fluid develops when, in the post-operative period, this fluid gathers in the deeper tissues. It is said to occur in between 0.07% and 2% of patients [2]. This is probably an underestimate if one considers the small symptomless pseudomeningoceles not infrequently seen on routine post-operative MRI studies.

A larger pseudomeningocele is eventually palpable as a soft fluctuant swelling in the wound. There is a danger that nerve roots will herniate into the cavity causing sciatic pain (*Figure 7.1*). If sacral roots are trapped in the cyst there is a serious risk to bladder and bowel function. Thus any patient who has a pseudomeningocele with nerve root symptoms needs a primary closure and repair before the neurological problem becomes irreversible.

> ***Case Report 12:*** *Worse after surgery*. Mr GS was a 52-year-old school teacher who had a spinal decompression for right root entrapment syndrome. During the operation the dura was torn. The dura was not sutured, but the surgeon wrote in the notes that a blood clot was left over the tear, and the wound was closed.

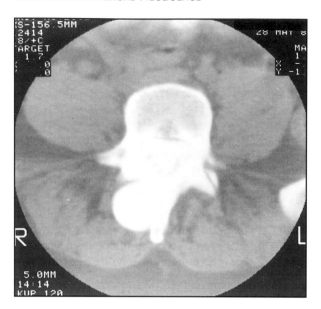

Figure 7.1. A CT myelogram of a patient with a right-sided pseudomenigocele which was causing pain in the back and leg.

Three weeks after the operation Mr GS had a lot of back pain and he noticed that the wound was swollen. He had headaches. He says that this was ignored when he attended the hospital follow-up clinic. The back pain increased, and he developed new symptoms in the left leg with urgency of micturition.

Four months after the operation he asked his general practitioner for a second opinion. He had an MRI scan which showed a small psuedomeningocele. It was thought that nerve roots were intermittently trapped in the neck of the sac. He had a surgical repair, but unfortunately his symptoms remained.

He argued that the dural tear should have been repaired and that in any event the Quekenstedt test should have been applied to the dura at the end of the operation. He claimed that if the psuedomeningocele had been diagnosed and treated earlier, he would have avoided subsequent nerve root problems.

The defence successfully argued that it was acceptable practice not to repair the dura, and that the Queckenstedt test is not routinely applied. It was agreed that an earlier MRI scan should have been performed and that this would probably have demonstrated the pseudomeningocele. It was denied, however, that surgery would have been carried out prior to the development of neurological symptoms, because asymptomatic pseudomeningoceles are common. By the time nerve roots were becoming trapped in the neck of the cyst, the outcome with surgery would have been the same as his current status.

Although dural tears cannot always be avoided, meticulous surgical technique reduces their incidence and complications. In the post-operative period, surgeons should always consider a pseudomeningocele as a possible cause of recurrent root pain, ask about headaches and examine for a wound swelling.

ACCIDENTAL DURAL PUNCTURE DURING AN EPIDURAL PROCEDURE

In about 1% of epidural procedures the dura is accidentally punctured and some of these patients believe that their long-term symptoms are related to this accident. Epidural injections are performed most frequently for anaesthesia in obstetric practice. They are also used therapeutically by clinicians treating low back pain. Injected steroids can reduce dural and root inflammation in a patient with symptomatic disc protrusion and in root entrapment syndrome. It is also thought that the mechanical pressure of 40 cc of fluid might release adhesions.

The most common complication of puncture is headache. It occurs in 23% of patients having accidental puncture compared with 7% with no recorded puncture [3]. The causality is tentative, because many patients with accidental puncture may be influenced by the memory of the episode. The headache is postural and frontal. It may affect the neck and shoulders and be accompanied by auditory and visual symptoms and nausea. These symptoms do not always accompany accidental puncture, but when they do, they are usually reported within the first 2 days. The headaches usually resolve with time, but a minority continue with chronic symptoms.

REFERENCES

1. Stolke D, Sollmann W, Seifert V. Intra- and post-operative complications in lumbar disc surgery *Spine* 1989; 14: 56–59.
2. Hadani FG, Knoler N, Tadmor R *et al*. Entrapped lumbar nerve root in pseudomeningocoele after laminectomy: report of three cases *Neurosurgery* 1986; 19: 405–407.
3. MacArthur C, Lewis M, Knox EG. Accidental dural puncture in obstetric patients and long term symptoms *BMJ* 1993; 306: 883–885.

Chapter
8

SPINAL INFECTION

Infection of the spine is fortunately quite rare. It can occur spontaneously or as a consequence of surgery. Post-operative infection can occur in the disc space as discitis, or in the superficial tissues as a wound infection. The post-operative incidence has been reported as between 1 and 5%. It can never be totally avoided, but the risk is reduced by adopting a careful operative technique. Serious consequences of infection can be minimized by having good post-operative care and a high level of suspicion.

IATROGENIC DISCITIS

The disc is avascular, and if organisms are introduced into the disc space by a surgical instrument or a needle, the body's defence mechanism is not very efficient. Without antibiotics its incidence after routine discectomy is up to 2% [1]. Some authors have shown a significant decline in infection to 0.6% with properly administered pre-operative antibiotics. It is not prevented by giving antibiotics during surgery, because there is a considerable delay in them entering the avascular disc space. Other surgeons rarely see post-operative discitis and do not give antibiotic prophylaxis at all. Much may depend on surgical technique.

Aetiology

Infection can be air-borne, with bacteria settling on the instruments or into the wound. It is reduced by using clean-air theatres, and keeping the number of theatre personnel to the minimum. Bacteria can enter the wound from the hands of the surgeon if a glove is torn, and if fingers are introduced into the operation site. A 'no-touch' technique reduced the incidence of infection considerably.

Clinical presentation

The diagnosis is often overlooked because of the variation in presentation. The signs of discitis are

- severe pain
- muscle spasm
- pyrexia, rigors, sweats (though they are sometimes apyrexial)
- X-ray changes are delayed

(i)   Pain must not be confused with the normal post-operative pain. It is usually more severe than would be expected, and it gradually increases in severity. The pain is usually intense, particularly when weight bearing.

(ii) As the patient stands up and walks, they also have a lot of muscle spasm. It causes a classical hyperlordotic lumbar posture, or a trunk list to one side. Straight leg raising is usually limited on both sides by back pain.

(iii) Although many patients have pyrexia, with night sweats and rigors, sometimes they are afebrile.

(iv) Plain X-rays are normal in the first 2 weeks.

Thus, unless there is a high level of suspicion, the diagnosis may be missed. One must be careful not to label these patients with severe pain and an abnormal posture as having a psychological problem with an exaggerated response, simply because they are afebrile and have normal X-rays.

Some patients have a low grade discitis. They have an uneventful recovery from the operation, only to experience increasingly severe back pain some weeks later. There may then be a history of fever, sweats and chills. The pain is out of proportion to the clinical signs, and the back is usually stiff, perhaps with a lordosis or scoliosis.

Management

Any patient with these symptoms requires an early MRI scan, which is very sensitive for discitis within 3 to 5 days of the infection. MRI has a high overall accuracy. It can be done quickly without ionizing radiation, and it provides good morphological imaging (*Figure 8.1*). Technetium scanning is normally raised in the operative area after surgery, and it is helpful for the diagnosis of discitis only at a later stage. Plain radiographs show no change until the infection has been present for a few weeks, and then the disc height begins to reduce. The white blood count may not be raised but the ESR is typically high. Blood cultures are frequently negative. If a blood culture is not positive, the organism and its sensitivity can be identified by needle biopsy.

Treatment is by a period of bed rest followed by a plaster cast or polypropylene jacket, and several weeks of appropriate antibiotics [2].

Progress

Severe pain can last for weeks, decreasing over many months. The natural course is for slow spontaneous resolution over an average of 7 months (range 1.5 to 24 months) [3]. Some back pain usually remains permanently.

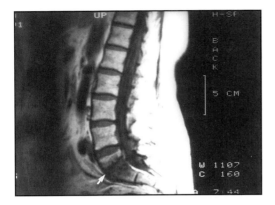

Figure 8.1. MRI of a patient with discitis at L5/S1. There is loss of disc space height and signal, with end plate erosions on each side of the disc (arrow). The decreased signal intensity on each side of the disc suggests osteomyelitis. The spinal cord can easily become compressed.

Occasionally the infection may progress to vertebral osteomyelitis, a para-vertebral abscess, or extension of infection into the epidural space.

Radiologically, the disc height reduces dramatically if the infection becomes established, and the adjacent bony margins become sclerotic. There is ultimately blurring of the end plate with end plate erosion. Advanced infection may show signs of osteomyelitis and para-vertebral abscess. There is spontaneous fusion at the level of the discitis in approximately 50% of cases.

Discitis must be accepted as a complication that can occur from time to time. A long delay in making the diagnosis, however, is not acceptable, and it increases the risk of long-term consequences.

EPIDURAL ABSCESS

This is fortunately a rare post-operative complication. However, it has a typical presentation of severe low back pain, fever, an elevated white blood count, and variable neurological signs. It is often associated with discitis or vertebral osteomyelitis. MRI is the most useful imaging modality, demonstrating the site and the extent of the abscess (*Figure 8.2*).

ARACHNOIDITIS

Arachnoiditis is an inflammatory intradural process leading to fibrosis which binds together the roots of the cauda equina. MRI, CT or myelography will show occlusion of the root sheaths (*Figure 8.3*), and sometimes concentric narrowing of the terminal theca. It may affect only one root. It is the result of intrathecal damage by surgical trauma, infection (bacterial, viral or fungal), foreign material, haemorrhage, steroid or anaesthetic agents.

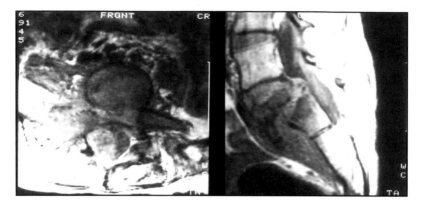

Figure 8.2. MRI showing an epidural abscess significantly compressing the thecal sac. The source of the abscess was discitis/osteomyelitis at L5/S1.

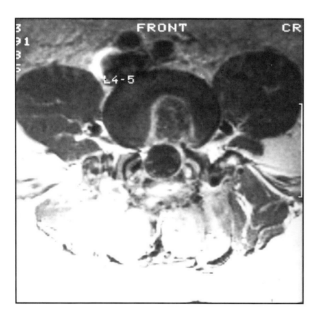

Figure 8.3. Arachnoiditis. Gadolinium enhancement shows nerve root sheaths clumping around the edge of the dura. It also shows a poor attempt of interbody fusion.

It is probably over-diagnosed as an explanation for failed spinal surgery when a patient has continuing back pain and discomfort in the legs for no apparent cause. It should not be mistaken for extradural scarring which is a common post-operative finding in aysmptomatic subjects.

It produces an aching and burning pain in the lower back, buttocks and perineum. Pain in a root distribution, although it may coexist, is probably from other causes.

WOUND INFECTION

Superficial wound infection is common and it usually responds to the patient's own defence mechanism. Deeper infection, however, can be troublesome.

Prophylaxis

Deep infection usually develops in a wound haematoma and therefore the surgeon tries to ensure that the wound is dry and that there is no dead space when closing the wound. Haematomas can not always be avoided. They are reduced by good surgical technique, and infection is avoided by evacuating a wound haematoma early. Two days of prophylactic antibiotics may reduce the risk of wound infection, but this is debatable.

Host factors which increase the risk of infection are

- increasing age
- steroid therapy
- poorly controlled diabetes
- chronic malnutrition
- immunosupression
- any remote infection.

These patients are at particular risk of post-operative infection and they should be carefully observed in the post-operative period, probably receiving prophylaxis.

Blood-borne infection may be inevitable, but to reduce its incidence, any remote infection should be identified and treated prior to spinal surgery.

Clinical presentation

Deep infection may be difficult to diagnose. The average interval between surgery and diagnosis is 11 days [4]. The wound can be deceptively normal. Patients complain of post-operative pain and generally feeling unwell, and they usually demonstrate pyrexia with raised white blood count and raised ESR. Imaging studies are not helpful. The diagnosis is confirmed by wound aspiration.

Treatment

When deep wound infection is diagnosed, the patient needs appropriate antibiotics. The organism and its sensitivity may be identified from a wound swab or, if there is a pyrexia, from a blood culture. It may be necessary to evacuate an abscess. A check should be made that the patient does not have reduced resistance as a result of another disease.

There should be no delay in diagnosis and treatment, because infection can track to the deeper tissues and ruin a good spinal operation. If there is serious infection in the presence of instrumentation, the metalwork usually has to be removed. Occasionally infection will induce septic shock with life-threatening consequences.

> **Case Report 13:** *Septic shock*. Mrs GL was a 63-year-old diabetic who had a spinal fusion with instrumentation at L4/5/S1. She was rather obese and unfortunately developed a haematoma in the wound which leaked and soiled the dressings in the first 48 hours after surgery. She had a pyrexia on the second day, and on the third day was distinctly unwell with a rigor. The operation had not been covered with prophylactic antibiotic, but on the third day a wound swab was taken and she was given Flucloxacillin.
>
> On the fourth day after surgery she was flushed, had a low blood pressure and a rapid pulse. She became confused and died of septic shock within a few hours.
>
> The surgeons were found to have mismanaged her condition. Death would probably have been prevented by proper care. They failed to recognize that an obese diabetic having instrumented spinal fusion was at considerable risk of infection. She was given no antibiotic prophylaxis. For 3 days she was not seen by any doctor more senior than a Senior House Officer. The risk of infection developing in the haematoma was not recognized. No blood culture was taken, and septic shock was not diagnosed until a few hours before her death. It was not defensible.

INFECTION WITH INSTRUMENTATION

The reported infection rate for spinal fusion is 0.7% to 11.6% [5]. The addition of instrumentation doubles the risk of infection. The infection rate without prophylaxis has been reported at 4.4% as opposed to 1.2% when antibiotic cover was used. Animal studies suggest that a single pre-operative antibiotic dose is as effective as antibiotics for 48 hours [5].

The pseudoarthrosis rate increases from 11% to 30% in the presence of infection. Thus, most surgeons will use prophlyactic antibiotics when fusing with instrumentation, although a minority of responsible surgeons will reserve antibiotics for obvious post-operative infection.

Infection has always been a hazard of surgery. It is now much less of a risk and, when it occurs, the surgeon is not usually to blame. However, there still needs to be great vigilance about prevention, diagnosis and management.

VERTEBRAL OSTEOMYELITIS

Vertebral osteomyelitis is most commonly caused by haematogenous spread of *Staphylococcus aureus*, although a wide range of other bacteria have been isolated, including coliforms, pseudomonas, streptococcus, brucella and *Mycobacterium tuberculosis*, fungi and anaerobes [6].

Infection of the spine is not easily differentiated from mechanical causes of back pain on clinical grounds alone. Infection may also be superimposed on a pre-existing back problem. Pain is aggravated by activity and relieved by rest. There is frequently a great deal of muscle spasm, more than is usually encountered with an acute disc lesion. However, the scoliosis of osteomyelitis is fixed, whilst in disc protrusion it is induced by standing up and abolished by lying down. There is usually pyrexia, loss of weight and loss of appetite, but all too frequently the diagnosis is not made until a late stage [7]. It may present as abdominal pain or be associated with other debilitating illnesses like diabetes. It should be considered in the elderly and in immuno-supressed patients.

Osteomyelitis of the spine can be demonstrated by bone scanning. It shows both increased uptake in the blood pool images as a result of increased blood flow in the affected bone, and also intense uptake in the later images (*Figure 8.4*).

Radiologically there is destruction of the end plate. The disc is soon involved and is rapidly destroyed by proteolytic enzymes of the pyogenic organisms. The infection spreads to adjacent vertebrae. Tubercular infection tends to spread to the next vertebra around the disc, and in spinal neoplasms the discs are generally preserved.

In children, haematogenous osteomyelitis affects the long bones. It is rare in the spine under 9 years of age, whilst the highest incidence is in the third decade.

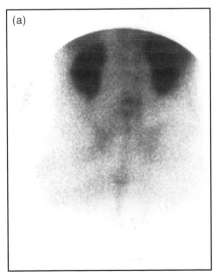
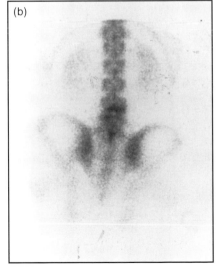

Figure 8.4. Bone scan of osteomyelitis of the lower half of L4 and upper part of L5 following disc surgery. **(a)** Blood pool. **(b)** Bone scan.

TUBERCULOSIS

Spinal tuberculosis, once quite rare in the UK is now appearing again. In previous generations it affected many vertebrae with collapse of the bodies and cold abscess formation. The discs were usually resistant to the infection. Cord compression from abscess formation, vertebral collapse or vascular involvement was feared (*Figure 8.5*). This picture is still seen from time to time, but more often it is encountered as an occasional disease of the elderly presenting much like pyogenic osteomyelitis. It is distinguished only by identifying the causative organism.

Surgery is necessary if there are neurological complications but, in the absence of spinal cord involvement, the only advantage of a radical operation is that it results in less late deformity than debridement. Chemotherapy on an outpatient basis has been shown to produce as good results as bed rest or a plaster jacket. Short-course antibiotic regimes are based on isoniazid and rifampicin which is as effective as 18-month regimes [8].

PRIMARY DISCITIS

This is an spontaneous infective inflammatory process which involves the paediatric intervertebral disc and the adjacent end plates. The most common organism cultured is *S. aureus*. The peak incidence is 6 years of age. There is a low grade fever, and back or abdominal pain. The child refuses to walk. The

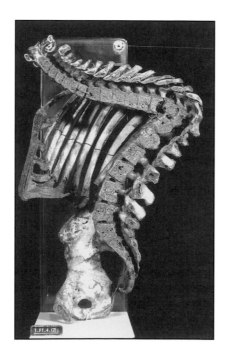

Figure 8.5. A skeleton from the museum of the Royal College of Surgeons of Edinburgh showing a marked thoracic kyphosis from a tuberculous abscess at T9–11.

ESR and white cell count are raised. The radiological features lag behind the clinical symptoms, though Technetium-99 bone scanning and MRI give a positive diagnosis at an early stage.

Although infection is quite rare in the spine, the surgeon should have a high level of suspicion for vertebral infection when the patient is distinctly unwell, when the appetite is poor and there is loss of weight, and when there is a lot of back muscle spasm. When these features are present, the possibility of infection must be considered.

REFERENCES

1. Stolke D, Sollmann W, Seifert V. Intra and postoperative complications in lumbar disc surgery *Spine* 1989; 14: 55–59.
2. Fraser RD, Osti OL. Discitis In: Findlay G and Owen R eds *Surgery of the Spine* Blackwell Scientific Publications, Oxford 1992; 631–635.
3. Lindholm TS, Pylkkanen P. Discitis following removal of intervertebral disc *Spine* 1982; 7: 618–622.
4. Keller RB, Pappas AM. Infections after spinal fusion using internal fixation instrumentation *Orthop. Clin. N Am.* 1972; 3: 99–111.
5. Guiboux JP, Ahlgren B, Patti JE, Bernhard M, Zervos M, Herkowitz HN. The role of prophylactic antibiotics in spinal instrumentation: a rabbit model *Spine* 1998; 23: 653–656.
6. Silverhorn KG, Gillespie WJ. Pyogenic osteomyelitis: a review of 61 cases *NZ Med. J.* 1986; 99: 62–65.
7. Flood BM, Deacon P, Dickson RA. Spinal disease presenting as acute abdominal pain *BMJ* 1983; 287: 616–617.
8. The 13th report of the MRC working party on tuberculosis of the spine. A 15 year assessment of controlled trails of the management of tuberculosis of the spine in Korea and Hong Kong *J Bone Jt. Surg.* 1998; 80-B: 456–462.

Chapter
9

UNCONTROLLED HAEMORRHAGE

Most spinal surgery causes minimal blood loss. There is not usually much bleeding from within the spinal canal, especially if patients are correctly positioned to avoid pressure on the abdomen. Disc surgery and spinal decompression does not usually require a blood transfusion. There is more bleeding during a spinal fusion when the cortex is removed from the posterior bony elements. Taking a bone graft from the pelvis may also cause sufficient blood loss to require transfusion. More serious bleeding is unusual, but sometimes the vessels external to the spine are in the operation field. There are one or two areas of potential danger.

THE AORTA AND INFERIOR VENA CAVA

In lumbar disc surgery major vascular injury is an unusual but life-threatening complication. One or two patients having spinal surgery in the UK each year will sustain an injury to the major vessels in the posterior abdomen. Vascular damage can occur when the surgeon is removing nucleus pulposus from the disc space. Mortality as high as 50% has been recorded [1]. Laceration of a major vessel may produce

- immediate haemorrhage
- an arterio-venous fistula
- a pseudoaneurysm.

Mechanism

The surgeon is frequently uncertain about how much of the nucleus pulposus to remove. Some argue that radical removal of the nucleus reduces the risk of another fragment extruding with further symptoms. A recurrence of disc protrusion will occur in 3–4% of patients. They may claim that this complication could have been avoided by a more radical excision.

Other surgeons favour a conservative approach, excising only the loose fragment and any other fragments which are loose in the disc space. They believe that more extensive removal of the nucleus pulposus is unnecessary, because the symptoms are caused by the loose fragment. Any nuclear material that is still attached will not extrude. Removing a lot of the disc will cause an inevitable reduction of the disc height, and this can have adverse late consequences. As the two vertebrae settle close together, the root canal becomes smaller with the potential for subsequent root entrapment syndrome.

The surgeon who is conservative in removing only the loose fragment(s) will not damage the great vessels. However, a radical clearance of the remnants of the nucleus pulposus from the anterior aspect of the disc does run the occasional risk of penetrating the anterior annulus with the disc rongeurs. This part of the operation is carried out blindly, by feel rather than by sight, as the rongeurs explore the anterior part of the disc space.

Most injuries involve the common iliac vessels during operations at L4/5. To avoid annular penetration extra care is necessary at this level, particularly in small patients because their discs are also small. Occasionally there is an anterior tear in the annulus through which the rongeurs can inadvertently pass. If the surgeon then grasps tissue with the jaws of the instrument, unwittingly the wall of the inferior vena cava or of the aorta may be damaged. The first sign of trouble is that there is blood on the jaws of the rongeur. The disc is avascular and the jaws should be clean.

Management of immediate haemorrhage

Once the surgeon suspects there may have been injury to the great vessels, the anaesthetist should be alerted and a large volume of blood ordered immediately. A vascular surgeon is called and the wound rapidly closed. If the patient is now showing signs of serious blood loss, no time should be lost in opening the abdomen and repairing the vascular defect. Prompt action can save a life.

One might argue that transecting the great vessels is an accident that could happen to any surgeon, though it might not be successfully defended. What is indefensible is procrastination in the management.

Case Report 14: Death after discectomy. Mr ST was admitted for a 'routine' lumbar discectomy at L4/5. Towards the end of the operation the anaesthetist noted that the blood pressure had fallen to 60/40 and there was a tachycardia of 140 per minute. The surgeon had noted some blood on the disc extractor and feared that there may have been damage to the great vessels. The patient was rapidly transfused with 1 litre of dextrose saline and three units of blood. In the recovery room his blood pressure improved to 70/50 and his pulse rate was still 140 per minute. The surgeon asked that four more units be prepared and that the patient should be closely monitored in the intensive care unit.

Two hours later Mr ST's abdomen was swollen and the blood pressure was hardly recordable. A vascular surgeon was called and theatre was urgently prepared, but resuscitation failed and he died on the operating table.

The claim of negligence could not be defended because the surgeon failed to recognize that the abdomen should have been explored immediately the great vessel damage was suspected.

Arterio-venous fistulae

Most reports in the literature are about arterio-venous fistulae [2] because of their unusual features. They may be missed initially because of limited external bleeding, and only about 10% are diagnosed within 24 hours. Some 20% are not recognized for more than 1 year [3].

Pseudoaneurysm

This is the least common sequel of vascular injury, and it may take a number of years for symptoms to become evident. Thrombo-embolism may be an important indicator of the diagnosis. There is one report of a pseudoaneurysm in the disc space [1].

ARTERIAL OR VENOUS BLEEDING DURING ANTERIOR SURGERY

The aorta and inferior vena cava are also at risk when operating on the lumbar spine from the front. These vessels, with their branches and tributaries, overlie the anterior aspect of the lower lumbar vertebrae and they have to be exposed and preserved during an anterior fusion. Sometimes, even when exercising great care, a tributary of the inferior vena cava is torn with troublesome bleeding. If it is not within the expertise of the spinal surgeon to repair the damage, the wound should be packed whilst waiting for the help of a vascular surgeon.

> **Case Report 15:** *Unjustified confidence.* Mrs TH was having an anterior spinal fusion, and during the exposure a tributary of the left common iliac vein was accidentally torn. The operation was being conducted by a senior orthopaedic trainee who was assisted by a trainee vascular surgeon. There was copious bleeding from the damaged vessel. Together they attempted a repair. After several failures, they requested the help of the consultant vascular surgeon. He successfully repaired the vessel. Post-operatively the patient developed considerable chronic swelling of the left leg resulting from deep venous thrombosis. The case was difficult to defend because of the inexperience of the surgeons and their delay in seeking expert help.

BLEEDING FROM THE SUPERIOR GLUTEAL ARTERY

The superior gluteal artery leaves the pelvis through the superior gluteal notch. It remains close to the iliac bone as it ascends deep to the gluteal muscles to supply the soft tissues of the buttock. It is at risk of injury when a bone graft is taken from the posterior ilium.

How damage can occur

The recommended incision to harvest bone from the posterior ileum follows the posterior aspect of the iliac crest and extends down over the upper part of the sacroiliac joint. The surgeon deepens the incision down to bone, incising the periosteum and then stripping the periosteum from the bone in a lateral direction. Provided the surgical exposure keeps close to bone and deep to the periosteum and does not transgress the gluteal muscles, and provided the superior gluteal notch is not exposed, the superior gluteal artery is safe. However, damage can occur if a retractor is placed in the superior gluteal notch in order to obtain a better view of the bone, or if the gluteal muscles are transected.

Management

If there is a sudden arterial haemorrhage and the vessel can be seen, the site is first packed for a few minutes to reduce the blood flow. The vessel is then exposed and ligated. If, however, the vessel can not be seen there is still a possibility that the bleeding will stop spontaneously. A vessel which is completely divided will contract and retract, and, in due course, stop bleeding. Therefore, with any sudden large arterial haemorrhage it is reasonable to apply a tight pack at the site and wait for a few minutes to see if it stops naturally.

When a vessel is only partially divided, however, it can neither retract nor contract and it continues to bleed. Potentially this is a serious vascular injury. The bleeding vessel needs to be identified and ligated.

If the superior gluteal artery is damaged as it leaves the pelvis through the superior gluteal notch it is difficult to visualize through a posterior incision. It tends to disappear into the pelvis and is not easily exposed. In this situation it must be identified from the front, and the spinal surgeon should call for the assistance of a vascular surgeon. The spinal wound is closed, the patient turned over and the bleeding vessel is identified in the pelvis.

Complications

It is important to treat this or any arterial injury seriously. A casual approach can lead to various complications

- massive loss of blood and haemorrhagic shock
- secondary haemorrhage
- late development of a false aneurysm
- haematoma and abscess formation
- major infection with multiple organ failure.

> **Case Report 16:** *A false aneurysm.* Mr DW was a 63-year-old retired manual worker, having a posterior spinal fusion for chronic low back pain. Bone was being harvested from the posterior ilium when there was

arterial bleeding from the region of the superior gluteal notch. The surgeon correctly packed the wound tightly and waited for 5 minutes. When the pack was removed the vessel continued to bleed and the wound was again packed whilst the surgeon continued to remove bone from the iliac crest. He did not obtain as much donor bone as he had hoped. He completed the fusion but left tight packs in the wound over the posterior ileum, to be removed a few days later.

No further bleeding occurred in the first 3 post-operative days, but when the packs were gently removed on the third day, the wound continued to bleed. Mr DW was taken back to theatre and the wound re-packed.

The wound became infected with recurrent episodes of bleeding. Arteriography demonstrated that a leaking aneurysm had developed in the pelvic part of the superior gluteal artery, and this was eventually explored and excised by a vascular surgeon. The wound continued to discharge for several months and, in the long term, the patient had more back pain than before surgery. He successfully claimed that the vascular injury had been mismanaged, that the damaged vessel should have been identified and ligated by a vascular surgeon at the time of the first operation, and that some of his back pain was the result of the complication.

Although bleeding from major vessels is uncommon in spinal surgery, when it does occur it is potentially serious. It requires prompt action and sometimes help from a colleague.

REFERENCES

1. Tanaka M, Nakahara S, Tanizaki M. Aortic pseudoaneurysm in the L3–L4 disc space after lumbar disc surgery. A case report *J. Bone Jt. Surg.* 1998; 80-B: 448–451.
2. Franzini M, Alana P, Annessi V, Lodini V. Iatrogenic vascular injuries following lumbar disc surgery: case report and review of the literature *J. Cardiovasc. Surg.* 1987; 28: 727–730.
3. Jarstfer BS, Rich NM. The challenge of arteriovenous fistula formation following disk surgery: a collective review *J. Trauma* 1976; 16: 726–733.

Chapter
10

PROLAPSED INTERVERTEBRAL DISC

Excision of a lumbar disc protrusion is the most commonly performed spinal operation, about 9000 being performed annually in England. It is not surprising, therefore, that this operation is responsible for much litigation. There are many causes for patient dissatisfaction, including failure to provide sufficient information about risks and benefits, operating too early or too late, neglecting a cauda equina syndrome, operating at the wrong level or on the wrong side, poor surgical technique damaging the dura or a nerve root, or poor post-operative care with failure to identify a recurrent disc herniation or a post-operative haematoma.

PATHOLOGY

When a disc protrusion becomes symptomatic, there has usually been a long period of silent degenerative change, first with fissure formation. If there are multiple fissures, a loose fragment will develop and this causes a major alteration in the disc mechanics. Under relatively small loads, the fragment will be displaced posteriorly, tearing the inner annulus and causing a protrusion [1]. If the fragment displaces further the whole thickness of the annulus gives way and the fragment is extruded as a herniation (*Figures 10.1* and *10.2*).

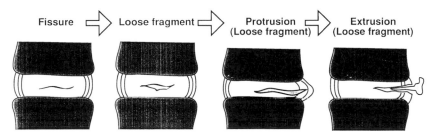

Figure 10.1. Diagram to show how a fissure can develop in a disc, and multiple fissures will produce a fragment. This is displaced posteriorly causing the annulus to bulge as a protrusion or tear extruding the fragment into the spinal canal.

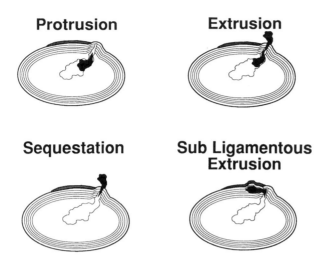

Protrusion

Extrusion

Sequestation

Sub Ligamentous Extrusion

Figure 10.2. A loose fragment of disc may cause a protrusion if the annulus is intact. The fragment may extrude partly into the spinal canal or completely sequestrate. Alternatively, it may pass under the posterior longitudinal ligament and remain sub-ligamentous and partly contained.

A protruding disc can compress a nerve root (*Figure 10.3*), depending on how much room there is in the spinal canal. In a large canal, the root can escape pressure. It is thought that the disc releases inflammatory mediators causing abnormality in the function of a compressed root. This is time-dependent, and although the disc may continue to compromise the nerve root, the inflammation can resolve and the symptoms settle.

CLINICAL FEATURES

The classical symptoms of lumbar disc protrusion are back pain and leg pain in a single root distribution below the knee. The leg pain is worse than the back

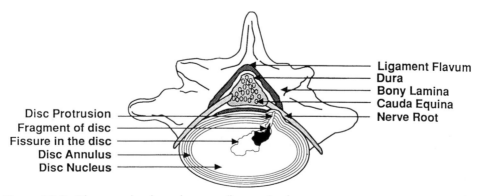

Ligament Flavum
Dura
Bony Lamina
Cauda Equina
Nerve Root

Disc Protrusion
Fragment of disc
Fissure in the disc
Disc Annulus
Disc Nucleus

Figure 10.3. Diagram to show how a disc protrusion can compress a nerve root.

84

pain. It is often made worse by coughing. The important abnormal sign is limited straight leg raising. This root tension sign is usually quite specific for a disc protrusion (*Figure 10.4*). If there is cross leg pain (*Figure 10.5*) – pain felt in the good leg when the symptomatic leg is raised – this carries a poor prognosis for conservative management. When straight leg raising is limited the patient usually volunteers that they have difficulty getting their socks on in a morning (*Figure 10.6*). About half of the patients with a disc protrusion will have a trunk list (*Figure 10.7*). There may be a reduced reflex, muscle weakness of wasting and sensory loss, but these are signs of nerve dysfunction and are not specific for disc protrusion.

Patients with disc protrusion present most commonly between 20 and 55 years of age, with a peak incidence at about 40 years of age. It sometimes occurs in children and adolescents. The presentation is a little different, with young people complaining less of pain and more of stiffness, with marked reduction of straight leg raising. The surgical indications are the same as for adults. They have a similar good surgical outcome [2].

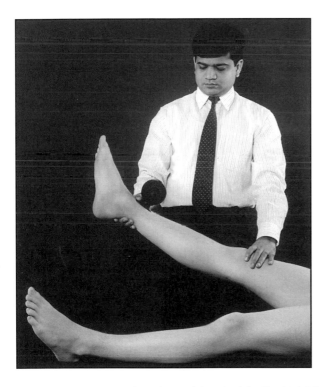

Figure 10.4. The straight leg raising test limited at 30°. It is a sign of root tension, a classical feature of a symptomatic disc protrusion.

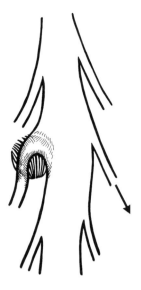

Figure 10.5. A diagram showing how tension on an asymptomatic nerve root can cause symptoms from irritation of a disc on the opposite side – cross leg pain.

INFORMED CONSENT

Patients need to be aware of the *natural history* of disc protrusion. Most patients with a symptomatic protrusion will get better without surgery. They may have back pain and sciatica as a result of root compression and inflammation, but 80% of patients with these symptoms settle down over a few weeks or months.

The patient who has 6 weeks of unremitting sciatica with limited straight leg raising which is not improving, needs to consider surgery. An operation is likely to produce a dramatic relief of the leg pain in about 90% of patients [3], getting them back to work in 3 months. Without surgery the recovery may be very slow, but in the long term – i.e within 5 years – there will be little difference between the operated and the non-operated patient. The only absolute indication for surgery is a cauda equina syndrome, producing bladder problems.

The patient considering surgery should know that the operation is designed to *relieve leg symptoms*, not back pain. Most can expect to be free of the leg pain quite soon after surgery, but 10% will continue with some slowly decreasing leg pain, probably because the nerve has been bruised by the protruding disc. Back pain will continue, varying in degree, for 65% of patients. A few (2–3%) will be worse as a result of unexpected complications such as nerve root damage, a dural tear and leaking cerebro-spinal fluid, and post-operative infection. If patients ask how they could be worse, the consequences of these complications are described. It is helpful if the surgeon writes down in some detail the conversation about obtaining informed consent.

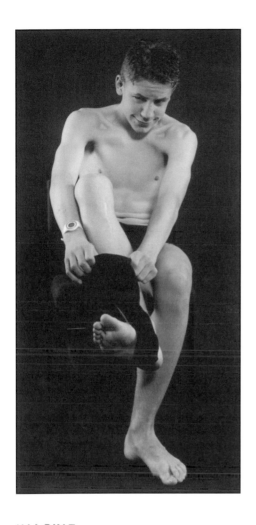

Figure 10.6. A patient who has sciatica and root tension has difficulty reaching down to the foot.

IMAGING

Imaging is essential to identify the level and the extent of the disc lesion. However, the diagnosis and the decision to operate is a clinical decision. It is not based on the results of imaging studies, otherwise one would operate on many patients with asymptomatic discs. When imaging shows two disc protrusions the clinical examination becomes highly relevant, because probably only one is symptomatic.

MRI

MRI will demonstrate disc protrusion in over 50% of the asymptomatic population. The purpose of imaging is to identify which level needs the operation, the topographical position of the disc (*Figure 10.8*) and whether there is any associated pathology like stenosis or an unexpected secondary lesion (*Figure 10.9*). MRI is now the imaging of choice for disc protrusion, being 97% reliable.

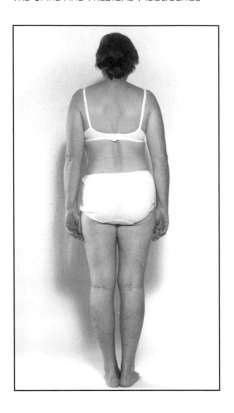

Figure 10.7. Photograph of a patient with a symptomatic disc protrusion causing a list to the left.

The high quality MR images now make it possible to identify whether the symptomatic disc lesion is a protrusion with a bulging annulus, or whether the annulus is torn with a sequestrated fragment in the spinal canal (*Figure 10.10*). If there is a sequestration, percutaneous therapy like chymopapain is not effective.

Myelography

Myelography will be positive in about 85% of protrusions (*Figure 10.11*). The disc protrusion is recognized by the 'cut off' sign when the protrusion indents the dura or compresses the dural sleeve of the exiting root. It is more accurate at L4/5 than at L5/S1, because the dural sac does not always extend down to S1, and the dural sac does not fill the spinal canal at this level.

CT scans

CT scans are 95% reliable but they involve ionizing radiation (*Figure 10.12*). A huge hernia can be missed on CT if it is not appreciated that the density of a massive hernia is different from the normal dura shown at another level (*Figure 10.13*).

Discography

Discography is not the best way to identify a disc protrusion but it is usually performed as a preliminary to chymopapain therapy, to identify the level of the lesion, to confirm the placement of the needle and, at the same time, to make sure that the disc fragment is not sequestrated (*Figure 10.14*).

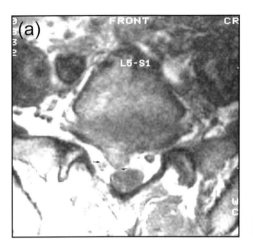 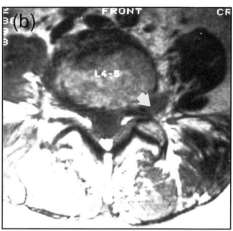

Figure 10.8. (a) MRI of a patient with a disc protrusion at L5/S1. The arrows show the disc fragment, medial to the nerve root. **(b)** MRI showing a herniated disc fragment at the intervertebral foramen.

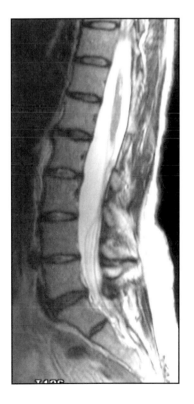

Figure 10.9. MRI of a patient with a disc protrusion at L5/S1 who also has a syringomyelia at T12/L1.

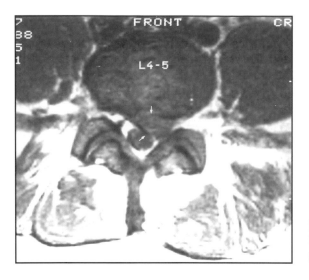

Figure 10.10. MRI showing a herniated fragment of nucleus pulposus.

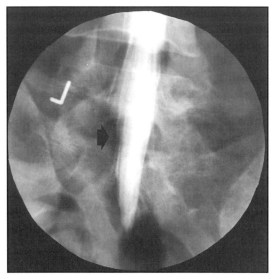

Figure 10.11. Myelogram of a patient with a left-sided symptomatic protrusion, showing the 'cut off' sign, where the nerve root does not fill with radio opaque dye.

THE TIMING OF SURGERY

There is a spectrum of different views about the best time to operate for a symptomatic disc protrusion. Some would argue that if symptoms and signs are not improving after 6 weeks, the patients should be encouraged to consider surgery. Others, aware of the propensity for disc symptoms to settle with time, and conscious that there are surgical complications, would recommend a longer period of conservative management unless there are socio-economic reasons why the patient needs to make a rapid recovery. Some patients who

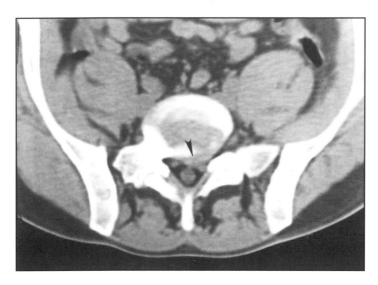

Figure 10.12. CT scan of a postero-lateral disc protrusion encroaching onto the nerve root.

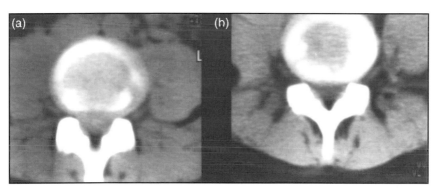

Figure 10.13. CT scan of a huge hernia **(a)**. It may be missed unless the density is compared with the normal dura at another level **(b)**.

have a poor result will sue their doctor for either being too hasty or too reluctant to operate. However, both the radical and the conservative views are acceptable.

There is a consensus about timing of surgery only when there is a cauda equina syndrome, or incipient cauda equina problems. It is agreed that in order to try to save the bladder function, emergency surgery is necessary, particularly in the partial cauda equina syndrome (see Chapter 6).

THE SITE AND THE SIDE

It is unfortunately quite easy to operate at the wrong level or on the wrong side. Every spinal surgeon has a policy to avoid this mistake, but the trend

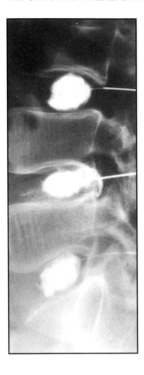

Figure 10.14. Lateral radiograph of discograms. L3/4 and L5/S1 are normal. At L4/5 the disc is protruding. The dye extends backwards but is contained by the posterior annulus.

towards smaller incisions and minimal invasive surgery increases the risk of mistaking the correct level. If the sacrum can not be confidently visualized at the time of surgery, then a radiological method must be employed to confirm the level of the lesion. Problems can occur if the fifth lumbar vertebra is sacralized or hemi-sacralized. At operation it is then found to be fixed and is misinterpreted as being the sacrum. L4/5 is then thought to be L5/S1 and a mistake is made in the segmental level.

The side of the lesion should be checked by the surgeon before each operation, and marked with indelible ink on the skin (see Chapter 19).

Case Report 17: *Wrong level.* Mr TP had surgery to remove a sequestrated disc protrusion at L4/5. He had temporary relief of leg pain whilst in hospital, but when he went home the symptoms rapidly recurred. He attended the follow-up clinic for several months, and eventually had further MR imaging. The surgeon told him that there was another disc protrusion and he should have another operation. On this occasion he developed post-operative discitis, with quite severe back pain and muscle spasm. His progress was slow and he requested a second opinion. It became apparent that the original operation had been at the incorrect level, and Mr TP then sued the first surgeon.

Operating at the wrong level is not defensible. However, the patient was unable to show that there was any loss, other than 8 months of pain and suffering, between the two operations. The discitis would probably have occurred if he had had surgery at the correct level, and his eventual outcome was no different to what it would have been if he had had correct surgery initially. It was settled out of court.

There was no excuse for the surgeon not telling Mr TP that there had been a mistake about the operative level when he had the first operation. A good doctor–patient relationship could have been maintained. Litigation might have been avoided and at least a frank explanation about the mistake would have enhanced the surgeon's reputation, whilst in effect it was diminished.

OPERATIVE TECHNIQUE

There are many acceptable procedures from microdiscectomy and minimally invasive surgery, to a more traditional fenestration. Much depends on the individual surgeon's experience. It is usual to blame the surgeon for poor surgical technique. Even when taking great care the dura may occasionally be torn, and leaking cerebro-spinal fluid immediately makes the operation more difficult. With gentle retraction, a nerve root may have its blood supply impaired, particularly if the pressure of the protruding disc has already disturbed the root circulation. The patient wakes up from the operation with more troublesome leg symptoms than before surgery, but this is a complication as a result of retraction and can not always be avoided. The assistant is advised to retract gently and intermittently, but still the root can be affected.

Damage to several roots is more suggestive of rough handling. Crushing of a root with a bone nibbler, or avulsion of a root with a disc extractor should not occur. This is more common if there are conjoint roots; with MR imaging duplication of roots can be recognized before surgery, and the risk of this root damage reduced.

Spinal stenosis makes it more difficult to visualize the nerve roots and remove a sequestrated disc, and, with this foreknowledge of a small spinal canal, the surgeon is usually prepared to make a larger fenestration or occasionally a hemi-laminectomy. There are no rules about how much bone should be removed in order to extract a disc protrusion. The surgeon simply ensures that he has good lighting and adequate vision.

Good pre-operative imaging will help the surgeon appreciate the extent of disc migration that can sometimes occur in a herniation. Foreknowledge makes sure that a fragment is not left behind. A fragment can migrate proximally or distally in the canal, or sometimes extend well into the root canal (*Figure 10.15*).

POST-OPERATIVE CARE

Most patients make a rapid and uneventful recovery from disc surgery, but occasionally a patient will have severe post-operative root pain which requires early repeat surgery. This is necessary if there is a further herniation of a fragment of disc, or if there is a post-operative haematoma pressing on the

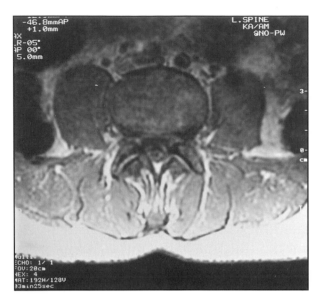

Figure 10.15. A large postero-lateral protrusion extending into the root canal.

cauda equina. Unless the surgeon is aware that a nerve root was damaged during the operation (when further surgery will be of no value), then early MR imaging will help to decide whether repeat surgery is appropriate. These patients need careful and thorough neurological assessment to know if there is a developing or a resolving problem.

INTRADISCAL PROCEDURES

- Chymopapain is an effective method of treating disc protrusion, but it is of little value if there is a herniation with the fragment extruded or sequestrated into the spinal canal. Many patients experience back pain and spasm for some weeks after the injection, but the long-term results, when compared with surgery, are encouraging [4].
- Percutaneous laser disc surgery and thermo-coagulation have not yet been properly evaluated.
- Automated percutaneous enucleation is designed to reduce the volume of the nucleus, but it has been shown to be of little practical value.
- Endoscopic discectomy is a difficult technique to learn, but if the fragment can be successfully removed, one can expect a good result [5].

These intradiscal procedures have their own risks. When approaching the disc percutaneously, it is possible to traumatize a nerve root, and to introduce infection (see Chapters 5 and 8). Chymopapain may also cause serious anaphylaxis if the surgeon is unprepared. In all of these procedures, the patient is warned that if they fail, surgery may be required.

POST-DISCECTOMY SYNDROME

This is a term used to describe a painful back after disc surgery, the mechanism of which is usually obscure. It may be the result of a low grade bacterial discitis, causing back pain and spasm. Curettage of the end plate at the time of discectomy might cause subsequent mechanical pain. Or the segment may be thought to be unstable, with un-natural movement causing pain. The facet joints might sometimes cause pain. There are no simple tests that will identify the cause of this pain and fusion is an uncertain remedy. Some North American surgeons suggest that post-discectomy syndrome can be reduced by incorporating a spinal fusion with the discectomy. This is not supported by the literature [2].

THORACIC DISC PROTRUSION

Thoracic disc herniation is uncommon, occurring with perhaps 2% of the incidence of lumbar protusions [6]. It is probably under-diagnosed. Many mild symptoms of thoracic pain may be related to thoracic discs, and asymptomatic protrusions are common. The aetiology is the same as for lumbar disc pathology, with disc degeneration and fragment formation. However, trauma may play a more important role than in the lumbar disc pathology, especially in young adults, because in normal every day life the thoracic spine is largely splinted and protected by the rib cage. When protrusion occurs, the pressure of the disc on the anterior part of the cord can have serious consequences.

The clinical features are variable. Many patients describe a dull thoracic pain for years with increasingly severe pain, often in a girdle distribution. If there is involvement of the spinal cord, there is progressive weakness, spasticity and numbness of the legs. Although the lesion is anterior, there may be posterior cord dysfunction with proprioceptive loss and an ataxic gait, whilst the motor power is well preserved. Urinary, bowel and sexual dysfunction are not uncommon. Because of its rarity and variable presentation, it is understandable that the diagnosis is frequently delayed. The differential diagnosis is tumours, demyelinating disease and infection. There needs to be a high level of suspicion. MRI will confirm the diagnosis.

There are various surgical approaches. The posterior approach, though traditional, is probably not the best. It is difficult by this method to remove an anterior disc in the thoracic spine. Although the postero-lateral approach does not give a very good field of view, it is appropriate if the disc fragment is lateral and not central. The anterior thoracic approach carries the risks of thoracotomy, but it provides excellent results with reports of 85% of patients either normal or improved. However, patients need to know that thoracic disc surgery carries a risk of serious complications. This needs to be balanced with the potentially serious natural history.

REFERENCES

1. Porter RW. Pathology of symptomatic lumbar disc protrusion *J. R. Coll. Surg. Edinburgh* 1995; 40: 200–202.
2. Papagelopoulos P, Shaughnessy WJ, Ebersold J, Bianco AJ, Quast LM. Long-term outcome of lumbar discectomy in children and adolescents sixteen years of age or younger *J. Bone Jt. Surg.* 1998; 80-A: 689–698.
3. Porter RW. Spinal surgery and alleged medical negligence *R. Coll. Surg. Edinburgh* 1997; 42: 379–380.
4. Cogan WJ, Fraser RD. Chymopapain: a ten year double blind study *Spine* 1992; 17: 388–394
5. Schreiber A, Suezawa Y, Leu H. Does percutaneous nucleotomy with discoscopy replace conventional discectomy? Eight years experience and results of herniated lumbar disc *Clin. Orthop.* 1989; 238: 35–42.
6. Russell T. Thoracic intervertebral disc protrusion. In: Findlay G and Owen R eds. *Surgery of the Spine* Blackwell Scientific Publications, Oxford 1992; 813.

Chapter
11

ROOT ENTRAPMENT SYNDROME

Root entrapment syndrome is a clinical term used to describe sciatic pain radiating down the leg in a root distribution as a result of root irritation from degenerative change in the root canal. The distribution of pain is identical to that from disc protrusion, but the cause is different.

PATHOLOGY

There is degenerative change from either bone or soft tissue thickening which reduces the available space for the nerve root. This may be in the lateral recess of the central canal where the root passes close to the pedicle before it leaves the canal at the next lower level, or stenosis may be in the root canal below the pedicle (*Figures 11.1* and *11.2*).

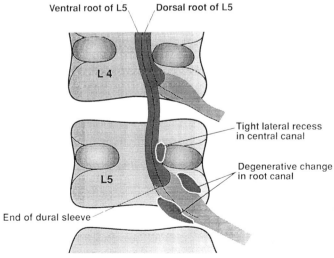

Figure 11.1. Diagram showing how the fifth lumbar root can be compressed by degenerative change in the lateral recess of the central canal or in the root canal.

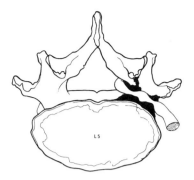

Figure 11.2. Diagram showing how degenerative change in the L5 root canal can compress the fifth lumbar root.

Thickened ligamentum flavum or fibrous thickening of a bulging degenerate annulus can restrict space for the nerve root (*Figure 11.3*). Root entrapment can occur in isthmic spondylolisthesis where osteophytes from a pars interarticularis can irritate a nerve root (*Figures 11.4* and *11.5*).

The nerve becomes thick and inflamed, but the neurological mechanism whereby the nerve becomes symptomatic, and why some compressed nerves are not troublesome, is not understood. Symptoms develop gradually and can become severe and unremitting.

MAKING THE DIAGNOSIS

Root entrapment syndrome causes pain in one leg in a root distribution below the knee. The pain in the leg is worse than the pain in the back. It develops

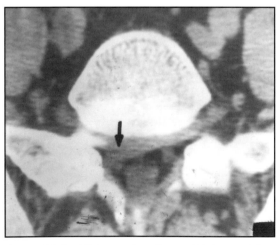

Figure 11.3. CT scan showing a thickened rim of bulging disc causing chronic irritation of a nerve root.

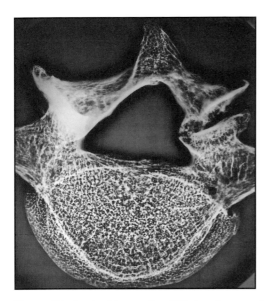

Figure 11.4. An X-ray of a fifth lumbar vertebra showing a unilateral pars defect. Degenerative change at this site is very close to the L5 root, and can be responsible for root entrapment syndrome.

insidiously and becomes severe and it is usually constant. The patient is usually over 40 years of age because degenerative changes are responsible for the root canal stenosis. These patients have pain in the same distribution as the patient with disc protrusion, but it is not made worse by coughing, it is not associated with a trunk list, and the straight leg raising is good. There are usually few abnormal signs.

The diagnosis is made clinically, and it is confirmed by imaging of the root canal by CT (*Figure 11.6*) and sometimes by MRI (*Figures 11.7* and *11.8*). Diagnostic root injection using radio-opaque material can demonstrate the course and degree of compression of a nerve root, and it is helpful to know if the pain is relieved after local anaesthetic injection. Because of false positives, this investigation is not considered a prerequisite to surgery. However, exploratory surgery without full imaging is no longer acceptable. The surgeon needs as much information as possible before operating.

INFORMED CONSENT

Most patients with root entrapment syndrome who see a spine surgeon have had pain for several months and it is quite severe. Decompression of the root canal is likely to relieve the symptoms, and surgery is therefore a reasonable decision. However, surgery is not mandatory and patients need to know that if they are prepared to wait, the sciatic pain will generally become less severe and over a few years it will probably settle down [1]. An epidural injection can

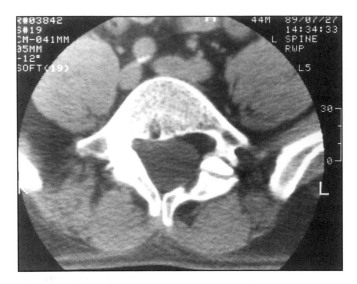

Figure 11.5. CT scan of a unilateral pars interarticularis which is irritating the fifth lumbar root.

help. However, most patients are not prepared to wait and are pleased to have a spinal decompression.

Therefore when symptoms are severe, and if they have been present for several months, provided imaging or diagnostic nerve root injections [2] support the diagnosis, decompression is appropriate. About 70% of patients can expect symptomatic improvement [3] with good results in the long term. A few (30%), however, will continue with root pain, and a minority will be worse.

MISTAKEN DIAGNOSIS

A decade ago, before root entrapment syndrome was recognized, patients with this problem were often misdiagnosed as having a disc protrusion. This is because the distribution of pain in both conditions is identical. In addition, patients with root entrapment syndrome may have imaging which shows a disc protrusion, because this is a common finding in the asymptomatic population. However, the protrusion may be innocent and not causing the problem. The clinical features of symptomatic disc protrusion, particularly the limited straight leg raising, are in contrast to those in root entrapment syndrome.

With a good history and a good clinical examination, root entrapment syndrome should not now be confused with disc protrusion. Removing an asymptomatic disc, and not decompressing the bony canal, will make the patient no better. This diagnostic mistake should not occur today.

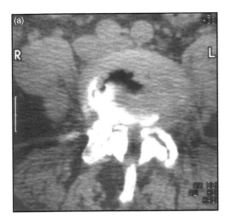
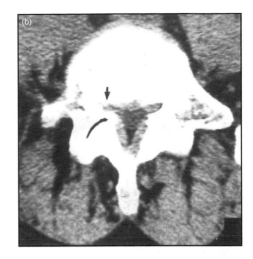
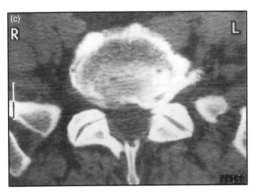
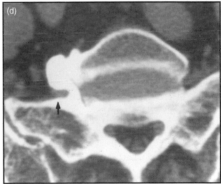

Figure 11.6. Spinal stenosis is readily demonstrated by CT. It may be **(a)** concentric central canal stenosis, or **(b)** in the lateral recess, **(c)** in the foramen or **(d)** extra-vertebral. The critical observation is flattening of the nerve root as in **(d)** and even then correlation with the clinical findings can be difficult and the patient may be asymptomatic.

THE OPERATION

When degenerative change is quite extensive and is at multiple levels, it may be difficult to be sure which root is pathological and at which site. The amount of decompression is then a matter of judgement. The surgeon tries to be conservative and avoid too much bony excision lest the spine become unstable, but if one is too conservative and decompresses only the root canal, it is possible to leave a more proximal tight symptomatic stenosis in the lateral recess of the central canal.

Patients with degenerative spondylolisthesis who also have root entrapment syndrome can develop further post-operative displacement with a recurrence

101

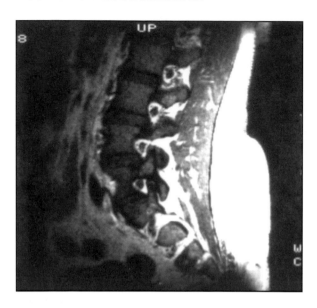

Figure 11.7. MRI showing normal intervertebral foraminae containing the nerve roots.

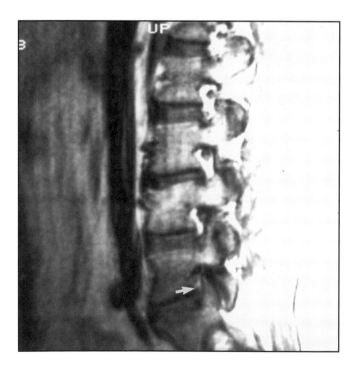

Figure 11.8. MRI with arrow showing subluxation of the superior facet of S1 into the root canal.

of symptoms. It may therefore be necessary to incorporate a fusion into the decompression. If there is marked degeneration, the displacement may have become stable and fusion is then less important.

COMPLICATIONS

- The root can be damaged. It is sometimes seen to be thickened and angry, and during surgery it is protected by a root retractor whilst the thickened bone is trimmed with a small osteotome. It is not always possible to visualize the root, and the root can be contused even by expert hands.
- Dural damage and infection can occur as in any spinal operation.
- Too much bone may be removed causing loss of support from the facet joints and subsequent post-operative spondylolisthesis.
- Too little bone may be removed and the root may not be adequately decompressed.

The operation can be difficult, depending on the degree of degenerative change and the presence of spinal deformity. There are no fixed rules about the extent of decompression, and the surgeon tries to make the best decision at the time.

REFERENCES

1. Porter RW, Hibbert C, Evans C. The natural history of root entrapment syndrome *Spine* 1984; 9: 418–421.
2. Stanley D, McLaren MI, Getty CJM. A prospective study of nerve root infiltration in the diagnosis of sciatica: a comparison with radiculography, computed tomography and operative findings *Spine* 1990; 5: 540–543.
3. Getty CJM, Johnson JR, Kirwan EO'G, Sullivan MF. Partial undercutting facetectomy for bony entrapment of the lumbar nerve root *J. Bone Jt. Surg.* 1981; 63-B: 330–335.

Chapter

12

SPINAL STENOSIS

Spinal stenosis is an anatomical term used to describe a small spinal canal. The canal reaches maturity in early life (*Figure 12.1*) and, if it fails to reach adequate size by 5 years of age, it will remain small throughout life. A trefoil-shaped canal is more troublesome than an oval-shaped canal. About 15% of adult spines have small trefoil-shaped spinal canals (*Figure 12.2*).

PATHOLOGY

Stenosis causes no symptoms unless the canal is compromised by other pathology. There are four pathologies that can cause problems if the spinal canal is already small:

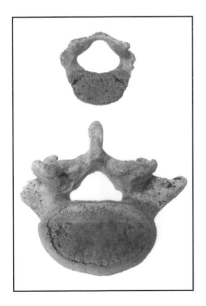

Figure 12.1. Photograph of an infant's fifth lumbar vertebra above, and an adult vertebra below. The infant's spinal canal is of adult size.

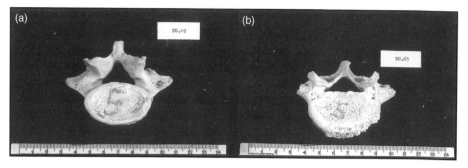

Figure 12.2. (a) A typical fifth lumbar vertebra with a large dome-shaped spinal canal. **(b)** A fifth lumbar vertebra with a shallow trefoil-shaped spinal canal.

(i)   disc protrusion encroaching into a small canal will produce more troublesome neurological symptoms and signs than would a similar disc in a larger canal;

(ii)   degenerative change can intrude into the canal, particularly laterally into the root canal, causing root entrapment pain;

(iii)   segmental displacement, such as in degenerative spondylolisthesis, will produce critical narrowing in a patient who already has spinal stenosis (*Figures 12.3* and *12.4*);

(iv)   multiple-level stenosis can cause neurogenic claudication. The cauda equina between two levels of stenosis becomes congested with venous blood which seems to impair the ability of the small arteries in the nerve roots to dilate during exercise (*Figure 12.5*).

CLINICAL PRESENTATION

(i)   Classical features of *disc protrusion* or *root entrapment* may be present without the clinician being aware that there is a degree of underlying stenosis. This is not apparent until the canal is imaged by MRI, CT or myelography (*Figure 12.6*). The images then show the added component of reduced space in the spinal canal. This will influence how the surgery will be carried out.

(ii)   If the stenotic patient escapes symptomatic disc protrusion and root entrapment in earlier life, they are at risk from *neurogenic claudication* in the more elderly years. Multiple-level degenerative change encroaches into the spinal canal (*Figures 12.7* and *12.8*), and these patients begin to feel discomfort in their leg(s) when walking. They have to stop for a rest, when the symptoms settle, but recur again each time the patients continue to walk. Symptoms are often worse when they walk down a hill because the spine is then in extension, and this tightens up an already small canal.

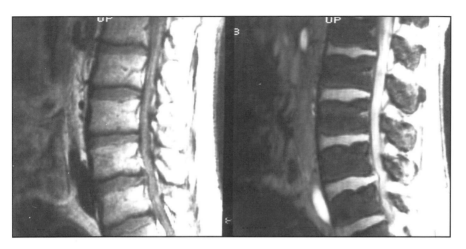

Figure 12.3. MRI of a patient with degenerative spondylolisthesis at L4/5 who also has spinal stenosis. There is not much degenerative change and if the spine is decompressed at L4/5 level, it would be sensible to also fuse the segment to prevent further post-operative displacement.

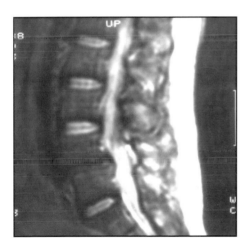

Figure 12.4. MRI of a patient with degenerative spondylolisthesis at L4/5. It is causing some stenosis. There is also some segmental stenosis at L3/4, with a thickened ligamentum flavum. The double level stenosis is causing neurogenic claudication. If the canal is decompressed there would probably be no need to include a fusion at L4/5, because with the degree of degeneration already present, there is not likely to be much more forward displacement post-operatively.

If there is a double level of central stenosis, all the cauda equina is congested and walking produces bilateral leg symptoms. If there is one level of central stenosis and a more distal level of root canal stenosis, one of the roots is congested with venous blood, and they have symptoms only in one leg (*Figure 12.5*).

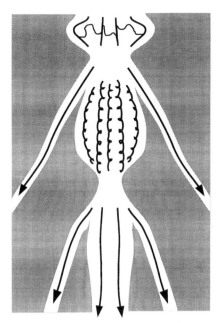 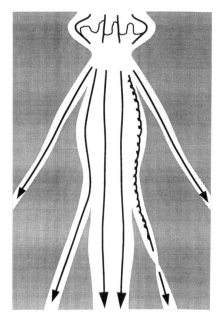

Two level central canal stenosis

Venous congestion of the cauda equina

One level central canal stenosis
and one level root canal stenosis

Venous congestion of one nerve root

Figure 12.5. Diagram **(a)** to show how two levels of central canal stenosis at L3/4 and L4/5 will cause venous congestion of L5 and the sacral roots giving bilateral symptoms. Diagram **(b)** shows a single level of central stenosis at L3/4 and root stenosis at L5 will affect L5 root and give unilateral symptoms.

MISTAKEN DIAGNOSIS

Before spinal stenosis was understood, and before MRI was readily available, patients with a block in the radiculogram at L4/5 were sometimes misdiagnosed as having a disc protrusion. The hour-glass constriction to the column of radio-opaque dye is very similar in appearance to that of a large central disc protrusion. The clinical presentation is different. The stenotic patient has back pain and problems with the legs when walking. The straight leg raising is good. Disc protrusion, however, gives root pain which is made worse by coughing. They have limited straight leg raising, and sometimes a trunk list.

The clue to diagnosing spinal stenosis lies in the radiculogram showing a 'canal full of roots' as the volume of injected dye is limited by the stenotic canal (*Figure 12.9*). It is no longer acceptable to misinterpret the radiculogram and operate on a patient with spinal stenosis, thinking that there is a disc protrusion.

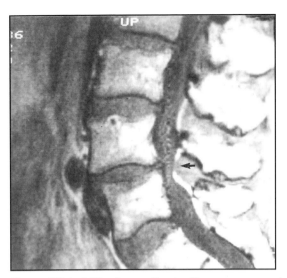

Figure 12.6. MRI of a patient with a narrow spinal canal and degenerative spondylolisthesis at L4/5 level. The thickened ligamentum flavum is compressing the canal from behind.

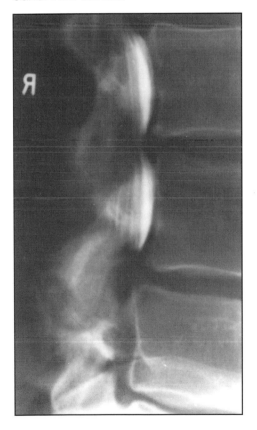

Figure 12.7. Radiculogram showing a developmental spinal stenosis, with a degenerative spondylolisthesis at L4/5 level and a second stenosis at L3/4.

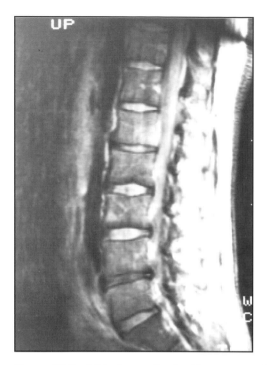

Figure 12.8. MRI of a patient with neurogenic claudication. There is developmental spinal stenosis (all the canal is narrow from L1 to L5) and in addition there is segmental narrowing at L3/4 and L4/5 from degenerative change.

THE SURGICAL IMPLICATION OF SPINAL STENOSIS

It may seem obvious that if a patient is having symptoms, and a small spinal canal is an important factor, then that canal needs to be widened by an operation. However, surgery is not essential, and it always carries a risk.

If the secondary pathology – the disc protrusion or the irritated nerve in root entrapment – will settle down conservatively, the need to operate can be postponed or avoided. The protrusion or the entrapment are treated in their own right and there is not an absolute indication for surgery. Although patients with neurogenic claudication do not get better, they do not necessarily get worse, and they need careful counselling about this natural history. Many are quite prepared to live with their disability if they know they are not likely to get serious neurology or go off their feet.

HOW MUCH BONE SHOULD BE REMOVED?

In previous years surgeons operating on spinal stenosis were much more radical, sometimes removing all the lamina at many levels. In the last few years surgery has become more conservative often with only a partial

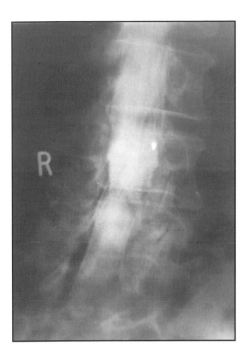

Figure 12.9. A myelogram of a patient showing some encroachment of the column of contrast medium at L4/5 level and outline of the nerve roots – a 'canal full of roots' typical of spinal stenosis.

laminectomy at the clinically symptomatic level. For example, when removing a disc protrusion in a stenotic patient, a total laminectomy is not usually necessary. A large fenestration is usually enough to decompress the nerve root and it reduces the risk of post-operative scar tissue compromising the root at a later stage.

In neurogenic claudication it was not uncommon to carry out a wide laminectomy and decompress five lumbar levels in patients. Now the current trend is to decompress only what is thought to be the symptomatic level by partial laminectomy.

Case Report 18: Too conservative. Mrs KH was a 48-year-old hospital secretary. She saw a consultant orthopaedic surgeon complaining that she had 8 years of increasing low back pain and 6 months of pain in the left thigh. The X-rays showed a degenerative lumbar scoliosis with 15° angulation between L3 and L5. A myelogram demonstrated some spinal stenosis at L3/4 and L4/5, and the CT scan showed quite marked bony thickening of the facet joints. After discussing the risks and benefits of surgery her name was placed on the waiting list for a decompression at L3/4/5.

Mrs KH was admitted to the hospital whilst her consultant was sick. The decompression was carried out by a senior trainee who was assisted by a more junior doctor. Mrs KH returned home after 12 days in hospital, but she says she was no better. The back pain and thigh pain persisted and she asked for a second opinion.

111

A new CT scan 18 months after the first operation showed only a narrow gutter of bony decompression at L3, L4 and L5 with the hypertrophied facet joints still encroaching into the spinal canal and compressing the dural sac (*Figure 12.10*). She had a further decompression by a neurosurgeon but still had no symptomatic improvement.

She claims that the first decompression was too limited, that the surgeon was inexperienced, and that a more radical procedure would have given a better result. She believes that by the time the correct procedure was carried out, the nerves were irreversibly damaged.

It was agreed that it was not good practice to allow a trainee to carry out what was obviously going to be a difficult operation without a consultant being scrubbed up and assisting. However, the defence successfully argued that the operation was probably carried out satisfactorily. They showed that there is a current trend for more conservative decompression. It was also recognized that bone can grow again and further compress a dural sac which was originally decompressed to a satisfactory standard. Studies show that there is no relationship between post-operative symptoms and the degree of decompression. Not all patients respond to a spinal decompression and there was unlikely to have been any irreversible damage to the cauda equina in the period between the two operations that would not otherwise already have been present.

SPECIFIC SURGICAL COMPLICATIONS

A stenotic canal can make the exposure of a disc protrusion somewhat difficult. The dura is pushed backwards against the ligamentum flavum leaving little extradural space, and when entering the spinal canal there is an increased risk of damaging the dura (*Figure 12.11*). Similarly, the lateral aspect of the canal may be difficult to visualize and when extracting the herniated disc the

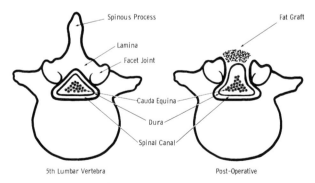

Figure 12.10. A diagram showing a central decompression of a spinal canal and the application of a fat graft to try to reduce the risk of post-operative scar tissue formation. The dura tends to bulge through the mid-line gutter. Undercutting of the facet joints would have provided a more acceptable degree of decompression.

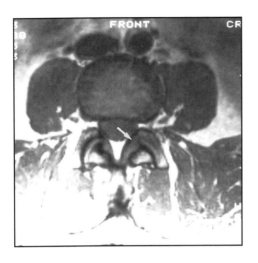

Figure 12.11. MRI with arrow showing the thickened ligamentum flavum. The facet joints are degenerate and the spinal canal narrow. The tightly compressed dural sac is at risk when decompressing the canal.

risk of root injury is increased. Making more space by excising more lamina than usual improves the exposure.

In neurogenic claudication the laminae are thicker than usual and have to be thinned with a drill, prior to nibbling them with rongeurs. During the procedure the dura can bulge dangerously through a narrow central gutter unless the surgeon is wary.

Patients with achondroplasia often develop spinal stenosis, and for these patients, decompression is particularly hazardous. The surgeon proceeds slowly and cautiously, using a dental burr rather than larger instruments, and there needs to be spinal cord monitoring in place lest there is damage to the lower cord (see Case Report 35, Chapter 19).

There is not really a risk of doing too little provided the decompression goes far enough laterally. Neither can a surgeon be criticized for doing too much. The amount of decompression is a decision which requires fine judgement and it is often made during the surgical procedure.

The spine can become unstable post-operatively with a gradual forward slip – a spondylolisthesis – causing a recurrence of symptoms. This can occur if more than half of the facet joints are excised, and particularly if there is already a degree of spondylolisthesis. Fusion at the time of decompression is then advisable. However, it is not always necessary to fuse a degenerative spondylolisthesis at the same time as decompression, provided there is a lot of degenerative change which has already stabilized that segment.

Patients with spinal stenosis who are considering surgery need to be informed about the underlying pathology and why stenosis is important. They need to know the natural history and if stenosis increases the risks of surgery. There is no doubt that when the surgeon operates with foresight, caution and skill, the results can be gratifying.

Chapter

13

SPINAL FUSION

Approximately 1200 lumbar spinal fusions are carried out in England each year. It is the third most common lumbar spine operation, there being 3000 decompressions, and nearly 9000 disc excisions every year [1]. Instrumentation for lumbar fusion has improved, but as the indications for fusion become clearer, it is probable that fewer fusions are now being carried out for low back pain.

INDICATIONS FOR FUSION

(i)   The most common reason for fusing the lower lumbar spine is *chronic low back pain* where the symptomatic pathology seems to be at one or perhaps two levels, and when all conservative treatment has failed. Unfortunately it is not possible to be totally sure that the fusion will be effective.

The surgeon can never be confident that the back pain is coming from a specific lumbar segment. If only one segment is pathological there is a better chance that fusion will help than when several discs are abnormal. Many surgeons will use provocative discography, injecting the radiologically normal and abnormal discs to make sure which disc space reproduces the pain. Unfortunately there are many false positives and false negatives which make the procedure rather unpredictable.

(ii)   However, spinal fusion has a good reputation for treating a painful *isthmic spondylolisthesis (Figure 13.1)*. Patients sometimes sue their doctor for delay in making this diagnosis, and for having to endure an unnecessary period of pain and suffering that could have been relieved by a fusion.

If there is marked displacement of S1 on L5 there is no doubt about the diagnosis of spondylolisthesis. However, only spondylolyisis may be present, with defects and no displacement. When there is only minimal

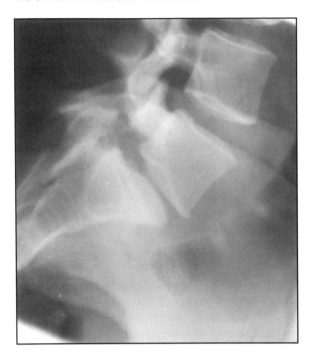

Figure 13.1. Lateral X-ray showing an isthmic spondylolisthesis at L5 with a forward displacement of L5 on S1.

displacement it can be difficult to visualize the lytic defects on either side of the pars interarticularis by standard antero-posterior and lateral X-rays. There may be a hint of the lesion because S1 is slightly displaced forwards and then oblique X-rays are necessary to show the defects (*Figure 13.2*). A CT scan may fail to demonstrate a defect unless the gantry is perpendicular to the table top [2]. One needs a high level of suspicion.

A defect may be present from early childhood but asymptomatic until there is some traumatic episode to disturb the fibrous union and produce pain. A period of rest from sport and perhaps a spinal support may encourage the defect to become stable again or even to heal. One can identify an acute strain to a pars defect (or even a stress fracture which may produce the defect) by bone scanning (*Figure 13.3*). If pain persist after a reasonable period of conservative management, a spinal fusion frequently produces a good result. Perhaps 80–90% of these patients will be markedly improved by a fusion, but one can not be so optimistic if there are signs of abnormal pain behaviour.

(iii) Fusion is sometimes advisable at the same time as a *degenerative spondylolisthesis* is being decompressed, if the decompression is likely to make the segment unstable. And it is appropriate when treating unstable *fractures, tumours* and *infection*.

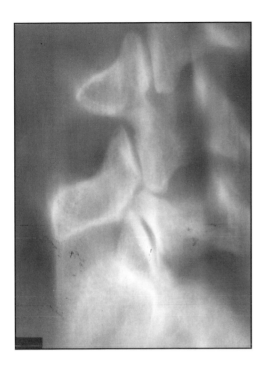

Figure 13.2. An oblique X-ray which is sometimes necessary to demonstrate a pars defect, if the lateral X-ray is not conclusive. The images should look like a 'Scottie' dog. The break in the neural arch gives the 'Scottie' dog image a collar.

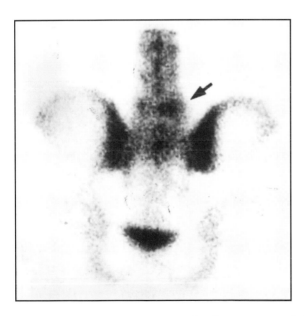

Figure 13.3. A bone scan showing increased uptake in the right pars interarticularis at L5 in a patient with acute pain from a spondylolisthesis.

117

The surgeon needs as much pre-operative information as possible. In the past, the pre-operative work-up has been a plain X-ray, and perhaps provocative discography (*Figure 13.4*) and a CT scan. Today, however, it is probably not good practice to fuse a spine without having an MRI. The excellent soft tissue images will demonstrate the state of the discs, the size of the spinal canal and the presence of any unexpected soft tissue pathology, like a spinal tumour.

CONTRA-INDICATION FOR FUSION

Sometimes patients are in great distress because of back pain and they put a lot of pressure on their surgeon to 'do something'. It is not good practice to offer a spinal fusion as a last resort because there seems to be no surgical alternative.

Abnormal pain behaviour is a strong contra-indication for fusion. These patients complain about low back pain but they have inappropriate features which warn the surgeon that there is an abnormality in the pain mechanism. The pain circuits in the spinal cord and in the brain remain active and are uninhibited. The patient feels the pain in the cerebral cortex. They are disabled but their complaints can not be explained in terms of organic pathology in the spine. If the major problem is not organic, then spinal surgery is not likely to help. In fact, it will probably compound the problem and make matters worse.

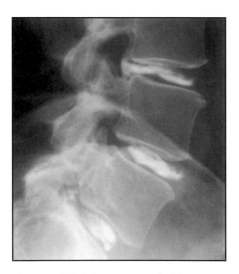

Figure 13.4. Discogram of L3/4, L4/5 and L5/S1. There is some degeneration at L4/5 and injection at this level reproduced the patient's pain. However, fusion at L4/5 alone would be unwise lest the grossly degenerate disc at L3/4 should later become symptomatic.

Inappropriate features are

- use of a stick, crutches, wheelchair
- wearing a collar and a corset
- slow movements
- staggering movements, though never falling
- needing help to dress and undress
- grasping movements
- keeping the eyes closed during examination
- low back pain to axial loading (*Figure 13.7*)
- low back pain to simulated rotation (*Figure 13.8*)
- excessive tenderness of the skin
- tenderness over the sacrum, sacroiliac joints and coccyx
- straight leg raising which is improved by distraction (*Figure 13.9*)
- non-dermatomal sensory loss
- inappropriate motor weakness.

A few of these signs are quite compatible with a normal response to pain, but when many are present, the patient is exhibiting abnormal behaviour. The patient genuinely feels the pain but, because of an abnormality in the pain mechanism, the source is no longer (or not much) in the lower back. To fuse the spine will be to court disaster, and the patient will be worse.

INFORMED CONSENT

When considering a fusion, patients need to be fully aware why surgery is being recommended. The principle of fusion for chronic low back pain is that pain is probably related to movement, and relief of movement at the symptomatic segment should relieve the pain (*Figure 13.5*).

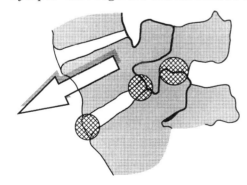

**Nociceptive source in structures
restraining SHEAR**
(muscles, ligaments, joint capsule, outer annulus.)

Figure 13.5. Diagram to show the possible sources of pain related to shear forces and segmental movement.

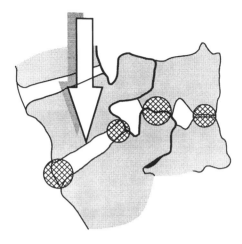

Nociceptive source in structures bearing load

(annulus, apophyseal joint, spinous processes.)

Figure 13.6. Diagram to show the possible sources of pain related to spinal axial loading.

The stakes are high. If the operation is successful, the patient is delighted. They are free of pain for the first time in years, and able to lead a fairly normal life style. This kind of result – a full recovery – although most gratifying to the patients and surgeon is not very common, and it can not be predicted. About 60% of patients having fusion for chronic low back pain will be improved to some degree by surgery but they still have some back pain. Some pain and disability remains, though they admit to benefit. However, the remaining 40% are no better and some are worse.

About 30% of patients are neither better nor worse. This is because

- the fusion is not sound, or
- the pain is not coming from the segment that has been fused, or
- the pain is related to loading of the segment and not to movement (*Figure 13.6*). Fusion does not remove the loading on a painful segment.

The remaining 10% are distinctly worse for having a failed fusion. This may be because the pain is coming from a higher level which is now bearing an increased strain. Alternatively, the fusion is not sound and there is a painful pseudoarthrosis. Or there may be a new psychological problem as a result of having major surgery which has failed. A minority suffer from a complication like nerve root damage, infection or donor site pain.

No responsible surgeon would fail to inform the patient of these risks, and ensure that they understand. It is useful to explain this also to a relative and

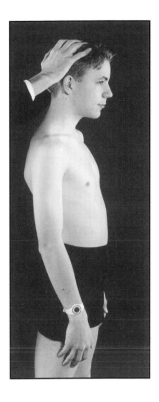

Figure 13.7. A patient being examined by axial loading. Pressure on the top of the head should not cause low back pain if there is a mechanical problem in the lower spine.

to record the conversation in the notes. When the risks and benefits are clearly explained to patients, many choose not to have surgery but to live with their pain, and this is probably the reason for fewer fusions now being carried out for low back pain.

Case Report 19: Failure to warn. Mrs JO'N was a 28-year-old self-employed dancing instructor. She had enjoyed an active life, horse riding and wind surfing, but had been troubled with intermittent low back pain for 5 years. When she was 25 years of age a consultant had told her that she had a degenerate disc at L5/S1. Physiotherapy had helped her temporarily. However, in the past 6 months the pain was constant and it was preventing her having a good night's sleep. She was having difficulty lifting. She could not do any sport and she was concerned that she might have to give up her business. The consultant told her that with this history and increasing disability, she would be well advised to consider a spinal fusion.

Mrs JO'N had a CT scan and provocative discography, and she says she was told that a fusion was likely to relieve her back pain, allow her to ride a horse and enjoy sport and maintain her job. She should be better in 3 months. She remembers being told that there was a 60% chance of being 60% better, but she does not remember ever being told that she could be worse after surgery.

She had a single level fusion at L5/S1 with pedicle screw and plate fixation. Any benefit was short lived, and 9 months after surgery she told her surgeon that she was worse than before the operation. She felt she was not being taken seriously and therefore sought a second opinion. This time she was told that she may have a pseudoarthrosis, or perhaps graft impingement on the L4/5 facet joints or maybe pain from a more proximal level. She agreed to have the metalwork removed and a further anterior fusion at L5/S1. She understood that there was now a 50% chance of improvement but she does not remember being told she could be worse.

After the further procedures she was still no better. She was in constant pain. She could not work and had to sell her business. Mrs JO'N is pursuing a claim for negligence, because she and her relatives are confident that if she had really been aware of the risks she would have declined the first spinal fusion.

Both surgeons say that they always tell patients that they can be worse after a fusion, though nothing was recorded about this in the notes. A written record would have given the surgeons better protection.

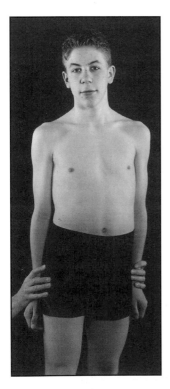

Figure 13.8. A patient being examined by simulated rotation. Turning the patient at the hips does not move the spine and should not be painful.

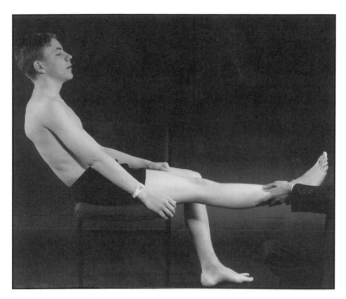

Figure 13.9. The 'Flip test'. After identifying limited straight leg raising on the couch, the patient is examined when seated by lifting the leg. If they flip over backwards the straight leg raising is genuinely restricted.

SURGICAL TECHNIQUES

There are many types of spinal fusion, with or without instrumentation, with an anterior or a posterior procedure or combined [3]. Bone graft may be autogenous from the patient's iliac crest, or a bone graft substitute can be used. All these various techniques are acceptable.

COMPLICATIONS

Nerve root damage from misplaced instrumentation will occur in spite of the surgeon taking great care. Infection must be accepted as an occasional complication, which increases the risk of pseudoarthrosis, and rarely settles until the metalwork is removed. The bone graft fails to unite completely in about 10–20% of fusions leaving a permanent pseudoarthrosis. The pseudoarthrosis rate is as much as 30% when infection is present [4].

Pseudoarthrosis may or may not be painful. It is not the result of faulty technique, and is a complication that must be accepted. Most surgeons will recommend a plaster jacket for 3 months after surgery if there is no internal fixation. However, the lumbar spine can still move by two-thirds of its normal range even when protected with a good external support. Not to provide a jacket is not poor practice.

Harvesting bone graft requires considerable care. The posterior iliac crest is the usual site for taking a bone graft when carrying out a posterior spinal

(a)

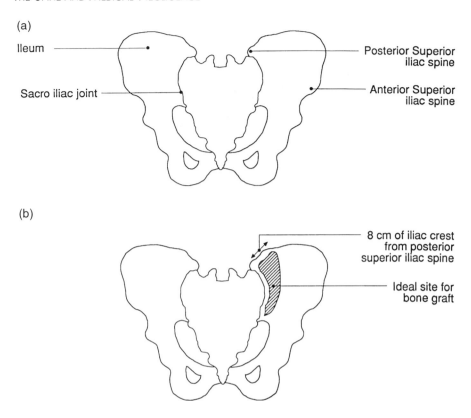

(b)

Figure 13.10. Diagrams showing **(a)** the anatomy of the pelvis and **(b)** the ideal site for removal of bone from the posterior ileum.

fusion (*Figure 13.10*). A separate oblique incision is made over the sacroiliac joint, and it is deepened down to bone.

The dissection should not extend as far down as the superior gluteal notch for fear of injuring the superior gluteal artery. Neither should the incision extend more than 8 cm lateral to the posterior superior iliac spine otherwise the cluneal nerves (the posterior primary rami of the upper three lumbar roots) may be injured. A post-operative neuroma on these nerves can be very troublesome.

Bone should be removed only from the outer table of the iliac bone. If the inner cortex is transgressed there is a risk of an incisional hernia.

> **Case Report 20:** *A pelvic hernia*. Mrs CF was 43 years of age, and had a spinal fusion for a painful spondylolisthesis. Bone graft was taken from the posterior iliac crest and, unfortunately, 6 weeks after surgery she developed an incisional hernia. A large painful swelling developed over the postero-lateral aspect of the iliac crest. It increased with coughing and straining, and there were bowel sounds on auscultation.

X-rays showed a large defect 8 cm × 6 cm in the posterior iliac crest 15 cm lateral to the posterior superior iliac spine (*Figure 13.11*). Although the original defect had been repaired (*Figure 13.12*), gas shadows indicated that there was now a large bowel hernia through the bony defect (*Figure 13.13*). Mrs CF required three attempts to repair the defect. The surgeon was unable to defend removing a full thickness bone graft at a site which was too far lateral.

It is unusual for surgeons to be sued because of a faulty technique when performing a spinal fusion. Complications do occur, and many patients have a poor result, but this is not usually the fault of the surgeon. More commonly patients sue because their expectations were too high. Their fusion fails to relieve the pain and they were not aware of this possibility. Failure to fully

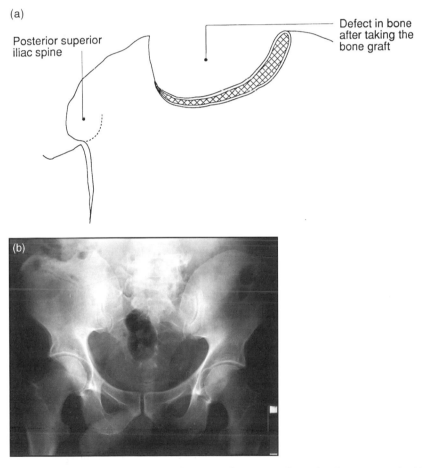

Figure 13.11. (a) Diagram to show an inappropriate site for removal of bone graft. **(b)** X-ray showing defect in the right iliac crest where bone has been inadvisably removed for a bone graft.

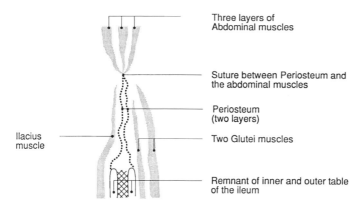

Figure 13.12. Attempted repair of defect.

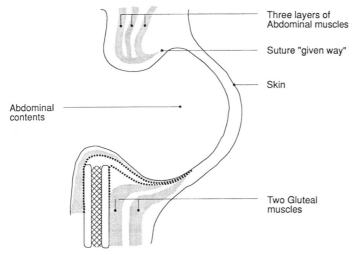

Figure 13.13. Subsequent hernia through the defect.

explain the uncertainty of the results of fusion is the major cause for complaint. It is here that surgeons need to be most vigilant.

REFERENCES

1. Okafor BE, Sullivan MF. Survey of spinal theraputic procedures in the United Kingdom *Eur. Spine J.* 1997; 6: 294–297.
2. Butt P. Radiological investigation of patients with back pain In: Porter RW ed. *Management of Back Pain* Churchill Livingstone, Edinburgh 1993; 101–113.
3. O'Brien JP, Holte DC. Simultaneous combined anterior and posterior fusion *Eur. Spine J.* 1992; 1: 2–6.
4. Lonstein JE. Management of postoperative spine infections In: Gustilo RB ed. *Current Concepts in Management of Musculoskeletal Infections.* Philadelphia: WB Saunders 1989; 243–249.

126

Chapter
14

FRACTURES OF THE SPINE

The most common fractures of the thoracic and lumbar spines occur as a result of a vertical compression force, sometimes combined with flexion, lateral flexion, rotation or extension. T12, L1 and L2 are the vertebrae most commonly affected, with decreasing incidence proximally and distally [1].

It is helpful to classify vertebral fractures in relation to the three columns of the spine: first, the anterior and middle parts of the vertebral body and the anterior annulus; second, the posterior cortex and posterior annulus; third, the posterior elements [2]. There are two important clinical questions when planning management [3].

- Is the spine stable?
- Is there neurological impairment?

PATHOLOGY

(i)   *Wedge compression fracture*. This is the most common vertebral fracture, resulting from an isolated fracture of the anterior column, following axial loading and flexion. There is usually no neurological deficit, but nerve damage can occur depending on the degree of kyphosis initially or in later years, and depending on the size of the spinal canal.

(ii) *Stable burst fracture*. Both anterior and middle columns fail as a result of a compressive load. If the posterior elements are intact (the neural arch), the spine is stable. Displacement of bony or disc fragments can compromise the vertebral canal causing neural compression. CT and MRI imaging tend to show that there is much more extensive damage than is apparent from a plain X-ray [4].

(iii) *Unstable burst fracture*. All three columns have failed. There is a tendency to kyphosis, with progressive neurological symptoms.

(iv) *Chance fracture*. This is a horizontal avulsion injury of the vertebral body following tensile flexion around an axis anterior to the spinal column.

(v) *Flexion-distraction fracture*. This affects all three columns following compression of the anterior column and tension of the middle and posterior columns.

(vi) *Translational injuries*. The spine is displaced in the transverse plane.

(vii) *Hyperextension injuries*. These account for less than 3% of spinal injuries. Disruption usually occurs through the disc with no bony damage to the anterior or middle columns. The posterior elements are usually comminuted with gross neurological damage [5].

(viii) *Fractures of the limbus*. Fractures of the rim of the superior or inferior margins of the vertebral bodies are not uncommon. They tend to occur in adolescents or young adults. They may be a small chip fracture, or involve more cancellous bone.

(ix) *Associated disc injury*. In addition to bony injury, the same forces can also damage a disc, either at the same site as the fracture or more distally. This is frequently missed clinically, being overshadowed by the more obvious fracture.

(x) *Damaged viscus*. Spinal flexion injuries can damage the abdominal viscera as well as the spine, particularly if the car seat-belt is misplaced across the abdomen rather than over the pelvis.

CLINICAL ASSESSMENT

The symptoms at the time of fracture may not be related to the severity of the compression [1]. The surgeon needs to be wary because a few patients with wedge compression fractures can remain on their feet. However, most have quite severe pain and tenderness at the site of injury. Retroperitoneal or mediastinal bleeding can be copious, adding to the discomfort. The extent of bleeding is best visualized by MRI.

Vertebral fractures are sometimes missed because of the severity of symptoms from other injuries. In resuscitation, clinicians rightly give priority to a head injury or thoraco-abdominal trauma, and the spine may be neglected, especially in an unconscious patient. A careful skeletal survey is therefore essential in the multiply injured patient.

Patients who fall from a height, landing on their feet, not uncommonly have a triad of bony injury – fractures of the heels, base of the skull and the spine. All three sites have to be examined (*Figure 14.1*).

A careful neurological assessment is essential. It may show normal neurology, or an incomplete or complete neurological injury at the level of the lesion. A changing pattern of neurology has management significance. A complete

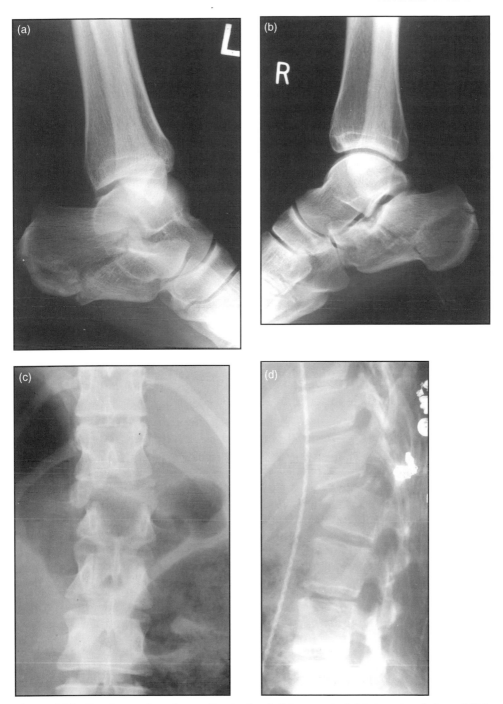

Figure 14.1. Radiographs of a patient who fell from a height showing **(a)** and **(b)** fractures of both heels, and **(c)** and **(d)** a flexion-distraction fracture of L2.

spinal cord or cauda equina injury that has not recovered at 48 hours is likely to be permanent [6]. Incomplete lesions in the thoracic spine can cause anterior cord damage whilst sparing some of the distal motor function and sparing the posterior column sensory positional and vibration sense. Less common is the central cord syndrome, with greater proximal than distal paralysis and varying degrees of sensory sparing. Rarely, a Brown–Sequard syndrome will give hemiparesis. Incomplete lesions have a potential for some recovery [3].

Imaging by plain radiographs will be insufficient if there is more than minimal radiological deformity and if there are abnormal neurological symptoms and signs. CT or MRI will then provide more information about the extent of the injury and its stability [7]. If there is any suspicion that the fracture may be unstable, the patient must remain in bed with very careful nursing, until further imaging confirms the stability of the spine.

Mistakes are sometimes made when assessing a thoracic spinal injury. It may be thought to be stable because the patient walked away from the scene of the accident, or because there may not be very much thoracic spine pain. If, however, there is a fracture of the sternum, or bilateral rib fractures in association with pain in the thoracic spine, it should be assumed that there is an unstable spine fracture until proved otherwise. An isolated fracture of a thoracic vertebra is usually satisfactorily supported by an intact rib cage. However, bilateral injuries to the chest wall with a fracture of a thoracic vertebra usually produce an unstable situation.

Case Report 21: *Unstable fracture.* Miss JD was a 23-year-old secretary. She was in the rear seat of a car which left the road in the early hours of the morning. She was found by the police and rescue services wandering around at the scene of the accident in a dazed condition. They thought she had been thrown out of the broken window of the car. She was taken by ambulance to the hospital and was smelling of alcohol. She had pain in the front and side of her chest, and was complaining of some neck pain. X-rays of the cervical spine were normal, but she had fractures of the ribs on the right, and tenderness of the sternum. She complained of tingling in her legs but there was no abnormal neurology. She was admitted for observation.

The next morning Miss JD still had unpleasant pain in her chest. She was encouraged by the physiotherapists to sit out in a chair and try to walk about in the ward. She was still complaining about her neck. It was mobile and not tender but she was given a collar.

In the afternoon she was again encouraged to get out of bed and she suddenly developed numbness below the trunk and weakness of her legs. She crawled back to bed. The houseman identified motor and sensory loss below T6 and organized an urgent X-ray of the thoracic spine. This showed a burst fracture at T5 and a CT scan identified a three-column injury. She was quickly referred to neurosurgeons who decompressed and stabilized the spine, but she was left with a complete neurological deficit at T6.

She claimed that an unstable fracture was missed, that she was allowed to mobilize and that this precipitated a complete spinal cord lesion which could otherwise have been prevented.

The defence admitted failing to diagnose an unstable fracture. They attempted to argue that there was an inevitable arterial thrombosis responsible for the sudden deterioration when she got out of bed, and that she would have developed the neurological problem in any event. A large settlement was ultimately made out of court.

MANAGEMENT

Stable fractures without neurological deficit

Patients with stable fractures and no neurological damage are usually advised to rest in bed until the reduction in the degree of pain allows mobilization with reasonable comfort. This may take a few days or a couple of weeks. Graded mobilization is encouraged to prevent the development of physical and psychological dysfunction. Many fears will be allayed if there is a careful explanation about the significance of the fracture. A good prognosis is expected and most patients in this category will become symptom-free. Should some pain persist, it is usually only intermittent and is not disabling. A temporary corset might help a mid- or lower lumbar fracture, but it does nothing to support a higher injury. Plenty of walking and swimming is advisable in the recovery period.

The degree of original kyphosis is probably related to the risk of a kyphosis subsequently increasing. If it is more than 40° it is likely to increase in the first 3 months [3]. However, there is no hard evidence that prolonged bed rest or that external support reduces the risk of a deformity increasing, if the fracture is otherwise stable.

Sometimes a CT or MRI scan will show that a large bony fragment has been extruded into the spinal canal, and it may appear to be compressing the neural elements (*Figure 14.2*). Provided there is no abnormal neurology or only slight impairment, and provided the spine is stable, surgery is not required. Remodelling can be anticipated over the next few years [8].

A neurological deficit

Decompressive surgery for complete neurological lesions has poor results whether performed early or late. However, many patients are offered surgery with a chance of neurological benefit. The surgery is generally helpful because the instrumentation will provide a stable spine with the opportunity for early mobilization in spite of the persisting neurological problem.

131

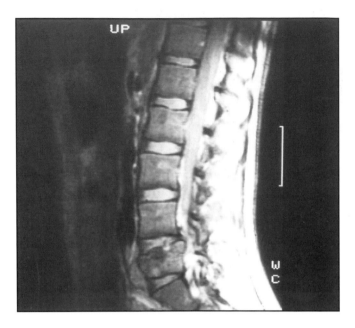

Figure 14.2. MRI of a burst fracture at L5 showing marked encroachment into the spinal canal. The patient had no abnormal neurological signs, and was treated conservatively.

Unstable fractures

There is a dilemma about the wisdom of surgery when the spine is unstable but there is no abnormal neurology or perhaps minimal deficit. Should the patient be treated conservatively, with careful nursing, until the fracture unites? Or is it preferable to operate and stabilize the spine? A stable spine will allow early mobilization, and perhaps reduce the possibility of further neurological problems. However, there is a risk of producing neurological damage by operating on a traumatized spine. The anatomy will be distorted, increasing the risk of incorrect placement of the metalwork (*Figure 14.3*). It requires a degree of experience and clinical maturity to make the correct decision, and it should be discussed with the patient and relatives.

> ***Case Report 22:*** *Discuss options.* Mr FH, a 46-year-old scaffolder, was admitted following a fall when he had a flexion-distraction fracture at T12/L1. It was a three-column fracture with some displacement, but there was no abnormal neurology. He was told that this should be treated with reduction, internal fixation and fusion, so that he could mobilize fairly quickly. The alternative was to spend many weeks in bed and, if there was then not a sound fusion, he would need later surgery. He and his family agreed.

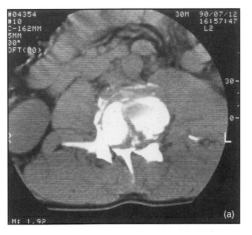

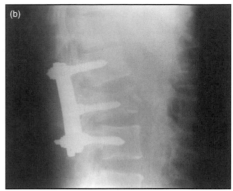

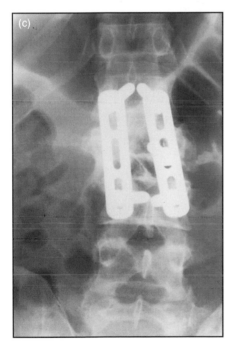

Figure 14.3. (a) CT scan showing an unstable burst fracture of L2. **(b)** and **(c)** Lateral and AP radiographs after internal fixation shows pedicle screws in what appears to be a good position. However, the screw at L2 was outside the pedicle and it caused serious damage to the conus of the spinal cord.

Unfortunately, because of the injury and displacement of the pedicle at T12, the pedicle screw was misplaced medially and it damaged the spinal cord. When he recovered from the anaesthetic he had asymmetrical motor and sensory loss in the lower limbs, and difficulty passing urine. This remained a permanent problem.

He and his family said that if they had been warned about any neurological risks they would not have agreed to surgical management.

There was no evidence that a conservative option had been discussed. It went to court and the defendants lost this case on the grounds of failure to obtain informed consent.

OSTEOPOROTIC COMPRESSION FRACTURES

These fractures are somewhat different to the traumatic fractures previously discussed. Osteoporotic fractures of the spine are very common in the elderly population, there being 15 new fractures per 1000 person years in white American women over 50 years of age [9]. In osteoporosis the bone density is reduced, but its quality is unchanged. It is reduced in strength, and with a moderate load the bone will fracture.

In an osteoporotic spine, a vertebral body may suddenly collapse during some normal everyday activity. Alternatively, several vertebral bodies may slowly collapse with a steadily increasing kyphotic deformity and some back pain (*Figure 14.4*).

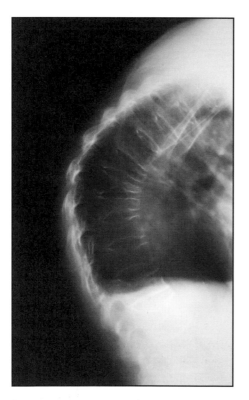

Figure 14.4. A lateral radiograph of a patient with a generalized thoracic kyphosis resulting from collapse of several vertebral bodies. Other causes of demineralization need to be excluded before this patient can be diagnosed as 'osteoporotic'.

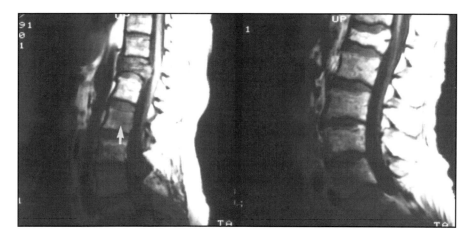

Figure 14.5. MRI of two patients. On the left there is compression fracture of T12 resulting from a metastatic deposit. There is a low signal intensity of tumour replacement on T1 images. The arrow shows a second metastatic deposit in an uncompressed L2 vertebra. On the right there is a compression fracture of L1 in osteoporotic bone. The bone has a higher signal intensity from fatty (non-tumour) replacement of bone.

Assessment and management

Patients whose kyphosis results from a steady insidious collapse of several vertebrae are usually seen at a routine hospital clinic. The diagnosis is straightforward and they may be given hormone replacement therapy. If, however, there is a sudden fracture of one vertebra, this can be quite painful. A careful assessment is needed to exclude other causes of demineralized bone such as bony metastases, osteomalacia (vitamin D deficiency), corticosteroid drugs, hyperparathyroidism, infection or a blood disease. These conditions can usually be excluded by a good clinical examination, but supplementary blood tests may be necessary, and sometimes MRI (*Figure 14.5*).

Most patients with osteoporotic compression fractures of the spine require only a few days in bed until the acute pain settles, and they can then mobilize again. Patients need to know that bed rest is to be discouraged because it increases the rate of demineralization, that a corset does not help, and that physiotherapy is not usually necessary. Failure to explain the mechanism and management of these fractures is sometimes responsible for anxiety and dissatisfaction, but litigation is not usually successful.

Case Report 23: *Osteomalacia.* Mrs QM was a 68-year-old shopkeeper who came from Pakistan 10 years before. She attended the Accident and Emergency department of a hospital complaining of sudden pain in her back. She was a little kyphotic and was tender at T7. An X-ray showed demineralization of the spine, a compression fracture at T7 and

135

compression of several other vertebral bodies. There was no sign of a primary tumour in her breast, thyroid or abdomen. She had been on no medication. She was told that she had an osteoporotic fracture, and that she should try to keep mobile, but avoid heavy lifting.

She continued to complain to her general practitioner about back pain and difficulty walking. He thought she might have arthritis of the hips, but this was not confirmed on X-ray. Two years later she had further X-rays of the hips which now showed radiolucent Lozer zones of the necks of the femora (*Figure 14.6*). This is a classical radiological sign of osteomalacia. Close inspection of the earlier pelvic X-rays showed that these Lozer zones were previously present, but they had not been recognized. She claimed that if osteomalacia had been diagnosed, she could have had vitamin D therapy with a better outcome. It was acknowledged that this diagnosis was missed both in the Accident and Emergency department and by the radiologist, and a settlement was made out of court.

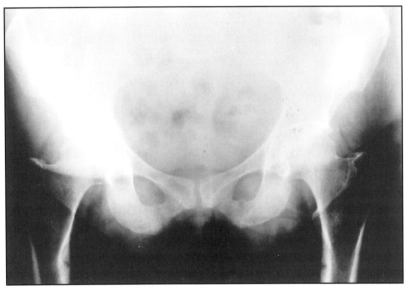

Figure 14.6. AP radiograph of the hips showing horizontal radiolucent areas in the medial cortex of the femoral shafts – Lozer zones – typical of osteomalacia.

REFERENCES

1. Young MH. Long term consequences of stable fractures of the thoracic and lumbar vertebral bodies *J. Bone Jt. Surg.* 1973; 55-B: 295–300.
2. McAfee PC, Yuan HA, Fredrickson BF, Lubicky JP. The value of computed tomography in thoraco lumbar fractures *J. Bone Jt. Surg.* 1983; 65-A: 451–473.
3. Bohlman HH Current concepts review: treatment of fractures and dislocations of the thoracic and lumbar spine *J. Bone Jt. Surg.* 1985; 67-A: 165–169.

4. Ballock RT, Mackersie R, Abitol JJ, Cervilla V, Resnick D, Garfin SR. Can burst fractures be predicted from plain radiographs? *J. Bone Jt. Surg.* 1992; 74-B: 147–150.
5. Denis F, Burkus JK. Shear fractures – dislocations of the thoracolumbar spine associated with forceful hyperextension (lumberjack paraplegia) *Spine* 1992; 17: 156–161.
6. Holdsworth FW. Fractures, dislocations and fracture dislocations of the spine *J. Bone Jt. Surg.* 1970; 52-A: 1534–1551.
7. Kerslake RW, Jaspan T, Worthington BS. Magnetic resonance imaging of spinal trauma. *Br. J. Radiol.* 1991; 64: 386–402.
8. Klerk LWL, Fontijne WPJ, Stijnen T, Braakman R, Tanghe HLJ, Linge B. Spontaneous remodelling of the spinal canal after conservative management of thoracolumbar burst fractures *Spine* 1998; 23: 1057–1060.
9. Cooper C, Melton LJ. Vertebral fractures *BMJ* 1992; 304: 793–794.

Chapter
15

SPINAL TUMOURS

PATHOLOGY

Bony tumours

Tumours are occasionally responsible for back pain. Secondary vertebral metastases are the most common of the bony tumours, with the breast, prostate, thyroid and kidney as the main primary sites. Primary bone tumours of the spine are unusual though Paget's sarcoma, chordoma, osteoid osteoma, angiosarcoma, solitary myeloma, malignant lyphoma and reticulum cell sarcoma can occur.

Bony tumours tend to affect the cancellous bone of the vertebral bodies and pedicles. They tend to give symptoms before there are bony changes evident on X-ray. A technetium bone scan can give presumptive evidence and determine the level and the number of the lesions (*Figures 15.1, 15.2* and *15.3*). MRI scans, however, will provide more information about the extent of the tumour in the spine and the soft tissue extension (*Figures 15.4* and *15.5*), and sometimes identify a benign diagnosis (*Figure 15.6*).

Small osteolytic deposits of multiple myelomatosis can be scattered through many bones causing back pain and fractures associated with these or with leukaemic deposits will cause pain.

Intramedullary tumours

These tumours occur in the spinal cord or the cauda equina. They may be extramedullary, like neurofibromas or meningiomas, or intramedullary, like ependymomas or astrocytomas.

DIAGNOSIS

Late diagnosis

Spinal tumours are frequently not diagnosed until a late stage. It can sometimes take years to make the diagnosis [1]. Unfortunately, this delay may

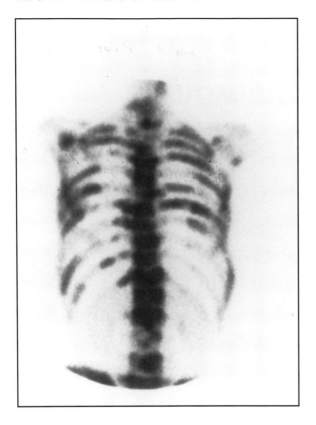

Figure 15.1. Bone scan showing widespread metastatic disease from a prostatic carcinoma.

affect adequate and optimal treatment and survival [2]. When patients complain about their management, this is usually because they think there has been unreasonable delay in making the diagnosis rather than any deficiency in operative or post-operative care. Why is the diagnosis difficult to make and why is it frequently delayed?

- Spinal tumours are quite rare compared with the high incidence of mechanical back pain. It is understandable that clinicians expect common conditions (*Figure 15.7*).
- Patients not infrequently attribute their first symptoms to a fall, suggesting an incorrect explanation for the pain.
- Spinal tumours generally present with back pain [1] the characteristics of which are indistinguishable from mechanical types of back pain. Like mechanical back pain, it is often aggravated by exercise though, classically, bone tumour causes constant pain.
- Degenerative pathology is so common in the general population that it is not surprising if spinal tumours and degenerative disease sometimes coexist. The surgeon may focus on a chronic degenerative back problem and miss the newly superimposed tumour.

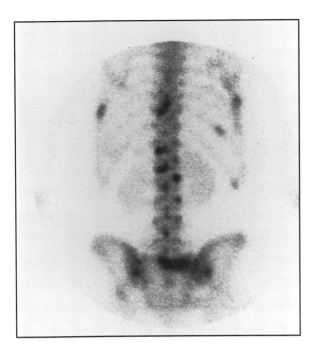

Figure 15.2. Bone scan showing multiple small metastases from a primary carcinoma of the breast.

- The diagnosis of a spinal tumour is frequently made from the bizarre neurological compressive symptoms, but unfortunately these features do not occur until a relatively late stage.
- X-rays do not show bony tumours until a late stage in the disease. Some intramedullary tumours can be missed on CT scan (*Figure 15.8*).

Clinical features

There are, however, a few features about spinal tumours that alert the clinician to this possible diagnosis. It is usually confirmed by appropriate imaging.

- A new symptom of back pain in an older person who has not previously had back pain, raises the possibility of a spinal tumour. However, this history alone does not justify the use of an expensive MRI investigation, unless there are other suspicious features. A screening ESR blood test is good practice. It would normally be raised in the presence of a tumour, but failure to carry out an ESR is understandable if other features support mechanical back pain.
- Pain from a spinal tumour may be intermittent and related to movement, much like mechanical back pain. However, if the pain is constant day and

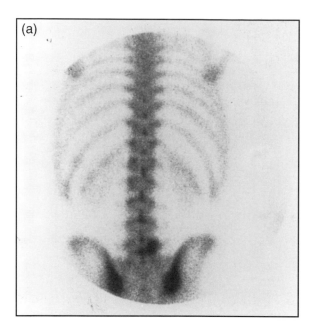

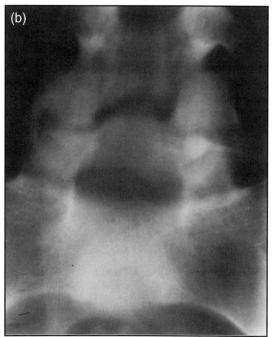

Figure 15.3. Bone scan of a patient with night pain and a very stiff spine. There is an osteoid osteoma of the right pedicle at L5. **(a)** Bone scan, **(b)** X-ray tomogram.

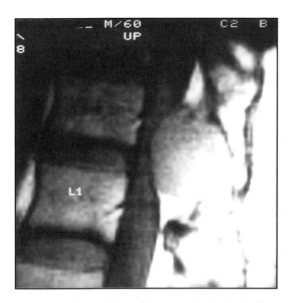

Figure 15.4. MRI showing a metastasis in the posterior elements at L1 from a renal cell carcinoma which was beginning to produce neurological symptoms and signs.

night and unrelated to movement, this is unusual in mechanical back pain, and tumour should be considered. Osteoid osteomas classically cause severe night pain.

- A spinal tumour tends to give steadily increasing symptoms, whilst mechanical back pain frequently fluctuates in severity, with exacerbations and remissions.
- Tumours may produce unusual neurological compressive symptoms such as numbness, tingling or burning with weakness and unsteadiness which can not be explained by a single nerve compression. If the lesion affects the spinal cord there may be a gradual development of spastic paraparesis, and bladder symptoms.

Although these tumours are rare, if the surgeon is to make an early diagnosis there needs to be a high level of suspicion [3]. Doctors acting for the plaintiff have to admit that it is regrettable, though understandable, that many of these tumours are not diagnosed until quite a late stage in their development

Case Report 24: *Delayed diagnosis.* Mrs KH was a 57-year-old house-wife, who complained to her general practitioner about back pain for 1 month. It was a new symptom and it was keeping her awake at night. It was constant and seemed to radiate round to her hips. She was referred to see a consultant who, after taking an X-ray, thought she had degenerative disc disease. She was referred for physiotherapy.

Two months later she was worse, with discomfort in her legs when she was walking. There were good quality hospital notes which also recorded

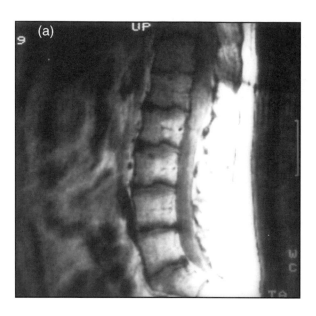

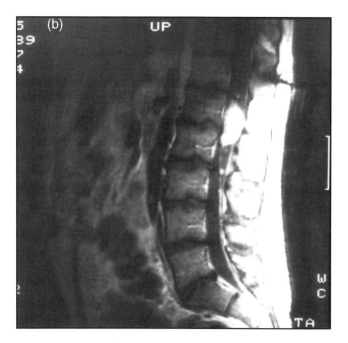

Figure 15.5. MRI of a tumour at the conus (the distal end of the spinal cord at L2) before **(a)** and after **(b)** gadolinium. It proved to be a schwannoma.

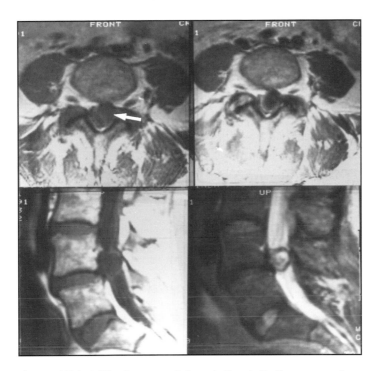

Figure 15.6. MRI of a synovial cyst. Top left: the arrow shows a cyst which is iso-intensive to CSF. Top right: post-gadolinium showing a surrounding halo which almost obliterates the thecal sac. Bottom left: there is a hyper-intensive rim noted after gadolinium injection. Bottom right: the hypo-intensive rim on T2 images is thought to be calcified or haemorrhage.

a stiff spine, some tenderness at L5 and no abnormal neurological signs. She had a lumbar MRI scan and was advised to have a decompression at L4/5 where there was some spinal stenosis. She declined surgery and sought a second opinion because she started to have unsteadiness when walking. Neurological assessment now showed sensory reduction below the waist, brisk lower limb reflexes and upgoing toes. An MRI scan of the thoracic spine showed a large neurofibroma at T11 which was promptly removed by a neurosurgeon.

She sued the orthopaedic consultant for delay in making the diagnosis. It was agreed that in retrospect one should have been suspicious about a possible tumour with a new onset of back pain, constant pain which became steadily worse, and a stiff spine. It would have been good practice to ensure that the first MRI scan included the thoracic spine. However, the absence of any abnormal neurological signs and with good quality comprehensive clinical records provided an acceptable defence that there was no mismanagement. There would have been a responsible body of

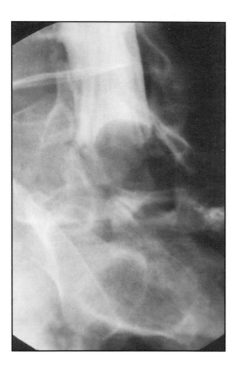

Figure 15.7. A myelogram performed for a patient with 4 years of back pain. It was performed prior to her being placed on the waiting list for a spinal fusion for isthmic spondylolisthesis at L5/S1. There is a large rounded filling defect which proved to be a rare paraganglionoma. When it was removed, it relieved her back pain.

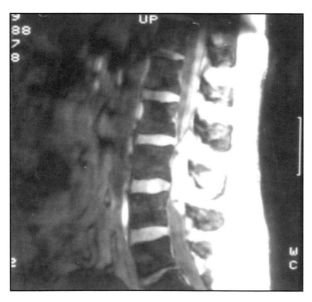

Figure 15.8. MRI showing a high intensity lesion in the spinal canal behind the body of L3. This lymphoma was formerly missed on CT scanning until the patient presented with paralysis.

clinicians who would not have investigated for a thoracic spine tumour until there were abnormal neurological signs.

REFERENCES

1. Weinstein JN, McLain RF. Primary tumours of the spine *Spine* 1987; 12: 843–851.
2. Weinstein JN. Spinal tumours In: Wiesel SW, Weinstein JN, Herkowitz H, Dvorak J, Bell G Eds *The Lumbar Spine* 2nd Edition Philadelphia: WB Saunders Company, Philadelphia, PA 1996; 917–944.
3. Findlay GFG. Metastatic spinal disease In: Findlay R and Owen R Eds. *Surgery of The Spine* Blackwell Scientific Publishers, Oxford 1992; 559–565.

Chapter

16

SCOLIOSIS

Scoliosis is a complex three-dimensional deformity with lateral deviation and axial rotation of the spine. It is troublesome mainly because of its cosmetic disfigurement.

TYPES OF SCOLIOSIS

There are several types of scoliosis:

- idiopathic adolescent scoliosis is the most common type. Its aetiology is unknown;
- congenital – when there is a structural abnormality of the shape of one or more vertebrae from birth;
- paralytic – such as in poliomyelitis or cerebral palsy;
- conditions affecting the spinal cord – such as syringomyelia or neurofibromatosis;
- infection such as tuberculosis;
- surgery to the thorax which can result in deforming contractures;
- infantile scoliosis is a deformity which can be present early in life with a potential to recover spontaneously;
- degenerative lumbar scoliosis. This occurs more frequently in women than in men, unusually after the fifth decade.

IDIOPATHIC SCOLIOSIS

This occurs more commonly in girls than boys. Its severity is measured from the angle subtended between the upper and lower vertebrae which have the most marked angular deviation (the Cobb angle). This does not take into account perhaps a more troublesome concern – the degree of rotation of the apical vertebra, which is the vertebra in the middle of the curve. This rotation can be very marked and, because the rib cage which is attached to the apical vertebra also rotates, there is a rib hump. Torsion is therefore a major cause of concern. The rib hump is the cosmetic deformity which most often concerns the patient (*Figure 16.1*).

Screening of normal school children has shown that a small degree of scoliosis occurs in 2–3% of the female population, and it tends to be unrecognized. This is because the rotational component of the scoliosis twists the vertebral bodies towards the convex side of the curve, but the spinous processes still tend to stay towards the mid-line. When viewing the spine from behind, it is the line of the spinous processes that is recognizable and this line does not seem to deviate until the curvature is quite marked. The mild rib hump is more noticeable than the curvature of the spine, and this is most noticeable when the patient bends down.

Scoliosis is detected by observing the child from behind. There is a lateral deviation of the spine, usually in the thoracic region, and the prominent rib hump. This rib deformity is exaggerated as the child flexes forwards, and this is how an early diagnosis is made.

Any child with a scoliosis should be referred to an orthopaedic surgeon with an interest in spinal deformity. Radiographs are taken, and the measurement of the Cobb angle is recorded. The child is usually asked to re-attend at

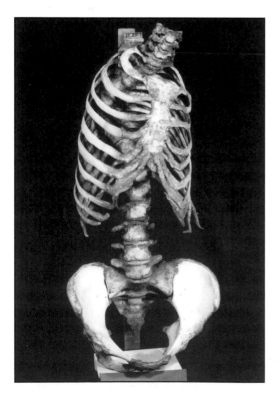

Figure 16.1. Photograph of a skeleton with idiopathic scoliosis. The thoracic cage is deformed in addition to the marked spinal deformity (acknowledgements to the Royal College of Surgeons of Edinburgh).

3-monthly intervals to determine if the curve is progressing. Repeat X-rays are taken at intervals of 3 to 8 months.

Progression

Curves of less than 10° are common, and clinicians will advise that children with this degree of mild deformity are merely observed until maturity. Most of these do not progress. When a curve is greater than 10°, there is a tendency for progression, and the earlier it presents, the greater is this risk. Such curves will usually increase with the adolescent growth spurt.

Double primary curves progress more severely than single curves. There is not usually much progression after the menarche. Curves tend to become stable once growth ceases. Cessation of spinal growth can be identified by the Risser sign – when, on an X-ray, the medial end of the iliac crest apophysis has ossified. Curves under 30° at skeletal maturity tend not to progress further, but thoracic curves of 50–80° at maturity, and lumbar curves can progress a little more in adult life (*Figure 16.2*).

MANAGEMENT

There are different views about management [1]. Some favour early surgery as soon as it can be predicted that a curve of 30–45° is progressing. This is to correct what tends to be seen as an unsightly cosmetic disfigurement. If the curve is allowed to become very severe, there will also be respiratory and

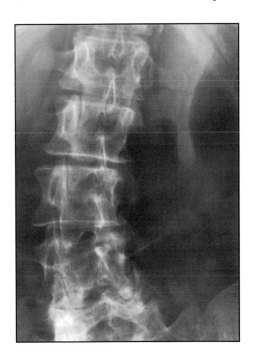

Figure 16.2. Antero-posterior X-ray of the patient with lumbar scoliosis. This tends to progress because of increasing degenerative changes. It will cause nerve root problems if the spinal canal is already small.

cardiac embarrassment. Other surgeons are less radical, believing that minor curves are not much of a cosmetic problem when compared with the possible risks of surgery, and they may allow a curve to progress beyond 45°. The deformity of the rib hump, which is the major concern, is not strictly related to the Cobb angle and therefore there are no fixed rules about when surgery should be recommended.

Pre-operative bracing is sometimes used in the hope of improving the final result of surgery. Different types of spinal braces can be used. The Milwaukee Brace is designed to be worn full time, apart from bathing and sport, but compliance is not good. Some methods of external bracing include skull halo-traction, but if a surgeon advises against the use of external pre-operative correction, this is acceptable.

The principle of surgery is to correct the deformity as much as possible with good instrumentation, and then fuse the spine in the corrected position with good quality bone graft. It is hoped that the fusion will prevent further progression. Once the fusion is sound after 3 to 6 months, the metal work has little further value, though it is left in place.

The operation must be done with the maximum degree of safety. In order to achieve these objectives a decision has to be made about the curves to be fused, the levels, the instrumentation and the surgical approach. It can be appreciated that the surgical technique to be adopted in any one particular child will depend to some degree on the surgeon's previous experience and training. Some favour a posterior approach with Harrington Rod instrumentation, sometimes with modifications by Cotrel or Luque. The anterior approach can use the Dwyer or Zielke systems. All are acceptable.

COMPLICATIONS

Neurological complications are the major surgical concern. Over-distraction is the danger, with a reported incidence of 0.2–0.8% of neurological deficits after surgery. Intra-operative spinal core monitoring has replaced the wake-up test to identify any operative damage to the spinal cord, but even when taking maximum care and releasing the correction if there are signs of cord dysfunction, neurological problems still occur. They are not the result of poor technique.

The complications common to all spinal surgery, such as haemorrhage and infection, are a possible risk when correcting scoliosis. In addition, the expectations of the parents and children about the cosmetic improvement should not be too great. The deformity will not be completely corrected. An unsightly rib hump may remain. Some of the initial correction may be lost. Parents and older children need to be aware of the limitations and risks of surgery.

> ***Case Report 25:*** *Unreasonable expectations.* Miss JF was 15-years-old and had idiopathic scoliosis. There was a single curve from T4 to T11 which had progressed to 55° over a 2-year period, and she also had an

unsightly rib hump. The risks and benefits of surgery were discussed and recorded. The operation was uneventful, and she had correction to 28°. When she was 17 years of age, the deformity had progressed again to 38° and the rib hump looked very unsightly. She agreed to have cosmetic surgery to remove the prominent angles of the ribs but a year later she was still very disappointed. She sued her surgeon because she thought she deserved a much better result.

The surgeon had not recorded that there might be a progression of the curve following surgery, nor that the surgery for the rib hump would not produce a perfect result, although it was always his practice to discuss these limitations. It was clear that the expectations of Miss JF were too high. It would have been better to make sure she understood the limitations of surgery at the outset, and to record this information, because although her claim did not succeed, it took a long time and much anxiety before there was a satisfactory outcome for the defence.

POST-OPERATIVE IMMOBILIZATION

Despite techniques to provide secure fixation, it appears that post-operative immobilization will enhance the fusion. It is not essential, but it is probably good practice at least with posterior fusions. External fixation may be with a cast or a brace. The model can be taken with the patient standing or supine, and the orthosis is worn day and night, with time out for showering. It is continued until the fusion is seen to be solid on oblique radiographs. Fusion may take up to 4 months, but on occasions it is twice as long. The post-operative activity level depends on the preferences of the surgeon.

It is never easy to be sure when fusion has occurred. Plain radiographs are unreliable, and CT is unhelpful because the metalwork scatters the images. Tomography can give an impression about the success of fusion, but only if the spine is explored again and the grafted area visualized, can the surgeon really know that the spine is soundly fused.

A Harrington hook can become disengaged in the early post-operative period. It is not necessarily the result of poor surgery, or because of unsupervized post-operative movement. Correction will have been lost and the hook should usually be replaced.

If a rod breaks, it tends to do so at a later stage. It indicates that the metalwork is under considerable stress and that the spine has not fused. It is not necessary to replace the rod if satisfactory correction is still maintained.

REFERENCE

1. Kostuik J. Assessment and treatment. Adult scoliosis In: Wiesel, Weinstein, Herkowitz, Dvorak, Bell Eds *The Lumbar Spine* Philadelphia: WB Saunders Company 1996; 1130.

153

THE CERVICAL SPINE

The spinal surgeon treats many cervical spine pathologies, from disc protrusion to degenerative stenosis, tumour, infection and trauma. Most of these conditions are managed conservatively, but occasionally surgery is required. There are a few litigation traps for the unwary.

WHIPLASH INJURY

This commonly occurs as a flexion strain to a passenger, when a stationary car is hit from behind. There is usually momentary pain at that time, and after a few hours the neck becomes stiff. Most clinicians now feel that, provided there are no abnormal neurological symptoms and signs, it is better not to use a collar but wait for a spontaneous resolution, perhaps with some physiotherapy. The symptoms can be expected to settle down over a few days or weeks, though they sometimes continue for many months.

Active treatment probably makes little difference to what should be a good natural history. However, the prognosis is less satisfactory when there are neurological features, if there is pre-existing marked degenerative change or if there is associated bony injury. Some of these patients, perhaps 19–42% [1] progress to have a chronic problem. Negligent claims occur when the doctor thinks there is only a whiplash, and neglects an underlying fracture.

CERVICAL FRACTURE/DISLOCATION

Bony injury to the cervical spine can be missed if the radiographs are not of good quality and if they are not carefully inspected. The lower cervical spine is a common site for bony injury, and depressing the shoulders whilst taking the X-rays ensures that this area is included in the lateral films.

If trauma to the upper cervical spine is suspected, odontoid views with the 'open mouth' X-ray is essential. A fracture of the odontoid process can usually be seen as a line across the dens.

Case Report 26: *Missed odontoid fracture.* JG was a 15-year-old boy who hurt his neck when he fell from a horse. He attended the Accident and Emergency department within 3 hours, complaining of a painful stiff neck. He was holding his head in his hands. The young casualty officer thought that routine X-ray films were normal, and JG was sent home wearing a collar. He was told to see his GP. He discarded the collar after a few days, and the neck stiffness gradually settled, but thereafter, whenever he headed a football his neck was painful. Because of mild continuing neck pain, he had a further X-ray a year after the injury, which now showed a displaced type-2 fracture of the odontoid (a fracture through the narrow portion where the bone is mostly cortical). He was referred to an orthopaedic surgeon who attempted to fuse the odontoid, but it failed to unite. He successfully sued the hospital where the fracture was missed on the first day, because the junior doctor had failed to notice the odontoid fracture which, in retrospect, could be seen as a distinct shadow.

It is good practice to treat an odontoid fracture with a halo-thoracic vest for 6 to 8 weeks followed by a firm collar for 4 weeks. Most fractures will unite in this period, but about 20% will remain ununited and will require surgery [2]. Non-union is more common in elderly patients and if there is a delay in diagnosis.

Dislocations with or without fracture are best reduced even if there are no neurological complications, but there is a spectrum of opinion about how this should be achieved [3]. Patients with a poor result sometimes sue their doctor for what they think was not the best treatment, but many different methods of management are practiced by competent doctors. These include

- halo vest (no surgery)
- non-halo orthosis
- posterior facet screws
- posterior wire(s) or clamp(s)
- anterior screw(s)
- traction until stable.

CERVICAL DISC PROTRUSION

Cervical disc herniation causing radicular pain or parasthesia is usually managed successfully with conservative treatment. However, the management of disc hernia with upper limb motor loss, or cervical cord involvement with slight lower limb symptoms remains controversial. The volume of herniated material often regresses [4], and surgery is therefore not essential.

When patients complain about surgery, they are concerned not usually about the technique, but failure to be offered a conservative option and failure to warn. Surgeons are now increasingly vigilant to inform patients that there are other treatment options. Even though disc surgery is usually successful, they may still be left with the same arm pain or muscle weakness. They could be worse if a nerve is damaged, and there is always the remote possibility of serious spinal cord damage by compression or vascular impairment. Failure to warn is not acceptable.

DEGENERATIVE DISEASE OF THE CERVICAL SPINE

Degenerative change in the neck is a normal phenomenon of ageing. However there can be three clinical problems:

- the neck may be chronically painful and stiff. This can sometimes be helped by regular physiotherapy;
- the foramen can be stenosed causing root pain and, if sufficiently severe, this may need decompressing, with all the risks common to discectomy;
- if the spinal canal is constitutionally narrow, the segmental degeneration can significantly compress the spinal cord at one or more levels and produce neurological problems in the legs. The patient becomes ataxic, with signs of an upper motor neurone lesion – brisk lower limb reflexes and up-going toes. The problem is likely to get worse unless the spinal canal is decompressed. Some improvement can then be expected, and at least further deterioration can be avoided.

Radiologists should be careful when imaging cervical spinal stenosis for fear that extension of the neck may permanently aggravate the problem.

Case Report 27: *Paraplegia after X-ray.* Mr SH was a 67-year-old man who complained of neck pain and a feeling of unsteadiness in his legs. There were no abnormal neurological signs. The clinician requested a myelogram of the cervical spine to exclude cervical spinal stenosis. When the radio-opaque material had been injected, he was lying face down on the X-ray table. He was asked to extend his head so that the films would show the maximum degree of stenosis. He then told the radiologist that his legs were feeling numb, but he says his neck was kept in the extended position. When he returned to the ward he had lost the feeling below C7, and had weakness in his legs. This partially recovered when he had decompressive surgery the following day.

He attempted to sue the radiologist. It was agreed that more care should have been taken of his neck, but his neck must have been very vulnerable. He would have had decompressive surgery once he developed abnormal neurological signs in any event and the outcome would probably not have been different

PHYSIOTHERAPY

Occasionally a physiotherapist will face litigation because a patient claims that they have symptoms as a result of their neck being inadvisably manipulated or treated with strong traction. It is essential that a therapist knows that neck pain is not caused by an underlying bony tumour or severe osteoporosis, because manipulation can then precipitate a fracture. Even though an early bone tumour may not be demonstrated on an X-ray, if there are any bizarre symptoms, the minimal requirement before manipulation is that the patient has had a recent X-ray.

Cervical traction has not been shown to be more effective at relieving neck pain than the natural history, but many individual patients believe it has done them good. It is therefore acceptable practice. Therapists are aware, however, that they must remove the traction if it is making the pain worse, and are cautious in treating the elderly.

REFERENCES

1. Freeman MD, Croft AC, Rossignol AM. Whiplash and associated disorders: redefining whiplash and its management by Quebec task force *Spine* 1998; 23: 1043–1049.
2. Stoney J, O'Brien J, Wilde P. Treatment of type-two odontoid fractures in halo-thoracic vests *J. Bone Jt. Surg.* 1998; 80-B: 452–455.
3. Glaser JA, Jaworski BA, Cuddy BG, Albert TJ, Hollowell JP, McLain RF, Bozzette SA. Variation in surgical opinion regarding management of selected Cervical spine injuries *Spine* 1998; 23: 975–983.
4. Mochida K, Komori H, Okawa A, Muneta T, Haro H, Shinomiya K. Regression of cervical disc herniation observed on magnetic resonance images *Spine* 1998; 23: 990–997.

Chapter
18

NEGLIGENT MEDICAL REPORTS

A clinician who is prepared to provide an expert opinion about personal injury must be able to defend this opinion against claims of negligence. Doctors acting on behalf of the plaintiff are particularly at risk.

EXAMINATION OF THE RECORDS

When reporting on lumbar spine problems the examining doctor is taking an unnecessary risk if X-rays of the lumbar spine are not examined. It is possible to mistake the diagnosis if one relies on the clinical examination alone.

> *Case Report 28: Mistaken diagnosis.* Mr GK was a 36-year-old labourer involved in a car accident. He was taken by ambulance to hospital complaining of pain in his back. He was told that an X-ray of the lumbar spine showed no bony injury. His back became less painful over the 3-week period that he was off work. When he was seen for the medical report 6 months after the accident the pain had largely settled. He was now able to keep at work, but did have some mild aching at the end of the day. The consultant said that he had had a mechanical strain to his back which was likely to resolve completely over a 12-month period, leaving no permanent problem. The claim was settled.
>
> Three years later Mr GK still had back pain, and he had given up his labouring job. Further X-rays had shown a spondylolysis at L5 and he was told that although this had probably been present for many years, the road accident had caused it to become symptomatic. He was considering a spinal fusion. He successfully sued the doctor who provided the medical report without examining the X-rays taken at the time of the road accident.

A doctor acting for the defence should not see the medical records unless the patient has given permission.

Case Report 29: Complaint to the GMC. Ms JD was a 35-year-old manageress. She believed that she had a disc protrusion from falling down stairs at work. A doctor was asked for an opinion by the defence and provided a report after examining her and considering a number of medical reports from several surgeons. Ms JD reported the doctor to the GMC because she thought he had examined her hospital and GP records without her consent. She was mistaken, and the GMC found no cause to take any action. It would have been helpful, however, if the doctor's report had clearly stated that the opinion was based on the clinical examination and on the other surgeon's reports, but on no other records.

THE SEVERITY OF AN INJURY

It is possible to misjudge the severity of an injury, especially when it involves structures other than the spine.

Case Report 30: Unrecognized renal damage. Mr WB fell from a ladder onto his back. He was taken to hospital in the firm's van. He was tender over the lumbar spine and an X-ray showed a fracture of the transverse processes of L2 and L3 on the left. He was admitted overnight and had microscopic haematuria. He was not investigated further. The back pain settled over 6 weeks and he returned to work. When he attended for the medical report by the defendant's doctor, 8 months after the accident, he was free of symptoms. The accident was thought to have been responsible for 2 months off work and a further 4 months of pain and suffering.

Two years later Mr WB saw an urologist with prostatism. An IVP showed that he had a non-functioning left kidney. There was no previous history of kidney trouble and it was thought that there had probably been unrecognized renal damage when he fell from the ladder. He successfully sued the doctor who reported on that injury, for failing to consider the possibility of permanent kidney damage.

ADMIT IGNORANCE

Doctors should take care when providing an opinion in an area where they do not have expert knowledge. It is always safer to acknowledge ignorance in areas outside one's own experience, and suggest that another opinion would be helpful.

Case Report 31: Sterility after a road accident. Mr KT was a 23-year-old factory worker who was thrown out of a car after a head-on collision late at night. He had a scrotal injury, fractured both superior pubic rami and the wing of the ileum, and had back pain. He was in hospital for a week and was off work for 3 months. At the time of the medical report the back pain had settled and he had no complaints. The surgeon said in the report that the accident had caused bony injury to the pelvis and a strain to the sacroiliac joints responsible for back pain which had settled over a period of 2 years. He also said that the accident had bruised the scrotum leaving no permanent problem.

Four years later the surgeon providing the report was sued because Mr KT had seen a doctor about sterility. It was alleged that the scrotal injury damaged his testicles. The defence successfully argued that it was highly improbable that the road accident was responsible for his sterility. However, the time involved in resolving this claim and the anxiety caused by the legal action was a high price for the surgeon to pay for failing to advise the solicitors to seek an expert opinion on the scrotal injury.

In a litigation-conscious society, doctors who profess to be expert witnesses will provide solicitors with a safe report if they do not provide opinions outside their field of expertise.

Chapter
19

RISK MANAGEMENT

WHY RISK MANAGEMENT?

Hospital management take a serious interest in medical negligence. This is partly because of its considerable cost, but the true costs of injury and litigation far exceed the immediate costs of compensation. The physical and emotional complications lead to an increased use of hospital resources [1]. Hospital staff are affected not only by the original incident but also by the ongoing process of litigation [2, 3]. It is a distressing and damaging experience, and one of the main sources of stress both for consultants and for over-worked junior doctors [4].

Every hospital needs a programme of risk management. The mounting financial cost of litigation makes this essential. The NHS executive has asked that providers take all possible steps to reduce claims for clinical negligence, and hence reduce costs, or at least moderate their expected increase [5]. Court awards are only a fraction of the total NHS expenditure on negligence claims [6]. When an 'accident' occurs patients usually develop huge and costly clinical needs. Litigation also engenders considerable administrative legal expenses for the hospital. And the health system also has a responsibility to recompense for unjust harm done to patients which our society currently sees in terms of money.

In any risk management programme the hospital needs to know the problem – what is its size, where the difficulties lie. There also needs to be an ongoing system for correction and education.

AUDIT

Each hospital should have in place a system of audit of previous and current claims for medical negligence and complaints. These should be continuously monitored. When the areas of risk are identified, there can be a corrective mechanism in place to 'close the loop' – audit, a change of practice and re-audit. There are several examples where audit will help.

Wrong level/wrong side

One of the most common problems responsible for high cost claims in spine surgery is operating at the wrong level or on the wrong side. Despite guidelines and long-standing efforts to avoid this problem, it is distressing that it still occurs. Two thirds of the claims for wrong site surgery are after orthopaedic procedures. It requires constant vigilance and ongoing education to ensure that there is a safe practice which eliminates this error.

At the time of admission the medical records should state the site and side of the planned procedure. It should also be recorded on the signed consent form. And this should be re-checked in the theatre immediately before the operation, both verbally with the patient, and from the records. The correct site and side are then marked with the surgeons initials. This mark should not be excluded from the operation site by theatre drapes [7].

Systems breakdown

Systems breakdown too often results in harmful errors. These may be:

- the administration of the wrong medication;
- the unavailability of appropriate instrumentation once the patient is anaesthetized;
- communication systems within the hospital failing at a critical time;
- office personnel not having been trained to permanently enter all laboratory and diagnostic data in the patient's records;
- scans not being available;
- lost correspondence;
- doctors not receiving messages and therefore failing to be in the right place at the right time;
- incorrect hospital records. A retrospective study of the accuracy of clinical records in patients with hip fracture at a prestigious teaching hospital showed that only 70% of the recorded data was reliable [8].

There are no easy or fail-safe mechanisms to eliminate these problems. Unfortunately, when a serious crisis occurs, it is often a summation of several small errors. Each may not be significant alone, but together they contribute to a disaster. Good quality audit needs to be in place in every hospital. This includes a careful and frequent assessment of all accidents and complications. Some problems are unavoidable, whilst others can be anticipated and avoided.

Audit will identify health care inequalities between hospitals, which may become the source of litigation in the future. We shall soon be in a position to know the national complication rates for various procedures, an encouragement to units performing well and an opportunity to correct poorer performance in others.

Electronic records

We have entered the era of paperless electronic records. This provides for efficient long-term storage of a large volume of data, both text and images, with rapid and accurate retrieval. Although this can reduce risk of systems failure, it also carries its own risk. The material is only as reliable as the person generating the input data, and it should be regularly assessed by audit.

EDUCATION

Aware of risk

When audit reveals areas of high risk, this information should be available for the whole clinical team. There is then an opportunity to prevent recurrences by education. For example, a surprising 42% of orthopaedic surgeons in North America had a poor understanding of proper ethical conduct with regard to informed consent [9]. Unfortunately, staff who are at risk may not be aware of their vulnerability, and they see no need to change their practice. Because allegations of medical negligence may occur relatively infrequently, staff at risk may be oblivious and unconcerned about possible claims. It is only after the event that they recognize the dangers. Thus, if litigation is to be reduced, there is a need for continuous education.

Which staff?

It is essential that the staff who are most at risk are aware of their vulnerability. Although no member of the hospital staff is exempt, it is the consultant specialist who is most frequently responsible for the high cost litigation in spinal surgery. This is followed by middle grade trainees, general practitioners, rheumatologists, anaesthetists and radiologists. Nurses, physiotherapists and para-medical staff can contribute to the litigation problems, although they are less commonly cited as defendants. The hospital management may find themselves at fault because of a systems failure, and failure to conduct and respond to audit.

Standard practice

There are areas where mistakes can be avoided by adopting a standard practice. Every member of the team should be aware of this policy. For example, a written policy will ensure that:

- one should never operate on the wrong patient if guidelines are followed;
- swabs will not be left in the wound if there is a double check of numbers of swabs prior to the closure of the wound, if a register of swabs used is maintained, if there are no loose swabs allowed in theatre, and if no swabs are removed from theatre without permission;
- there will be no systems failure of the anaesthetic apparatus if the check list recommended by Association of Anaesthetists of Great Britain and Ireland is observed [10];

165

- contemporary records are entered in the theatre operation-book about the patient, operation, timing, the name of the surgeon, assistants, anaesthetist and sometimes the instrument nurse.

Case Report 32: A retained swab. Mr PS attended his general practitioner over a period of 5 years complaining about low back pain. It seemed to be a typical mechanical back problem, with episodic pain which was made worse by exercise and relieved by rest. He was eventually referred to the hospital clinic and after many months he had an MRI scan. This showed an unusual soft tissue image over the sacrum. Forty years before, when he was in his teens, he had had surgery for a sacral haemangioma. The soft tissue lesion was thought to be a foreign body, and surgical exploration showed that it was an old retained swab probably left behind after being used to pack a bleeding wound. It was now encased in fibrous tissue. The current back pain was not thought to be related to this swab, but he successfully sued the previous hospital authority, whose policy for counting swabs at that time had failed.

Case Report 33: Awake during anaesthetic. Miss SF had decompressive surgery for root entrapment syndrome. She had the misfortune to be the last on the operating list [11]. The day after the operation she told the nursing staff that she had been awake during the procedure. She was distressed that she had felt the knife and the instruments in her spine. During the operation the anaesthetist had noticed that the anaesthetic gases had become disconnected for a short period, and wisely he had recorded this in the notes. He explained this to Miss SF and that she had been in no danger, and apologized for any distress she had experienced.

The operation to relieve leg pain was not successful and the sciatic pain remained. In addition she had nightmares, a personality change, and unnatural fears of hospital. It was agreed that the problem would not have occurred if the anaesthetist had adhered to the standard 'check list'. A settlement was made out of court.

Common errors

Audit will reveal that the areas which are responsible for most errors are:

- informed consent – not explaining the risks;
- operating on the wrong side or at the wrong level;
- operative complications such as nerve damage, csf leak, infection or vascular damage;
- surgery which is not sufficiently radical (i.e. too little decompression);
- surgery which is too radical (i.e. too much decompression);
- failure to relieve symptoms;
- a surgical or anaesthetic accident;
- primary surgery delayed too long;
- delay or failure to re-operate when the first result was poor;

- too hasty surgery;
- surgery carried out by an inexperienced surgeon;
- too many doctors.

Team education

Risk management means these common problems must be regularly addressed by every team conducting spinal surgery. They are primarily the responsibility of the consultant surgeon, who should make sure that they are routinely considered by the whole spinal team – that is, all the medical and para-medical staff who are in any way involved in the management of patients having spinal surgery.

Responsibility for the performance of the department, particularly organizational aspects, lies with the clinical director, in conjunction with the trust's management [12]. It should be the duty of the managers to check that there is an ongoing educational activity in every spinal unit to look at these specific issues. Because junior doctors change posts every 6 months, and other staff may be similarly mobile, it is sensible to have a 6-monthly rolling programme regularly discussing areas of specific risk. This should be seen not only as a method of reducing negligence claims, but also a means of establishing and maintaining a system of good clinical practice and high quality patient care.

> *Case Report 34: Too many doctors.* Mr. WK was a 33-year-old with a history of 8 years of chronic back pain after falling and possibly fracturing the sacrum. He had been a perpetual student for 10 years. At one time the pain radiated down the left leg, with limited straight leg raising, but back pain was his main problem.
>
> He was referred to a hospital of excellence. He was first seen by a research registrar who arranged for him to have physiotherapy. At his next visit he saw a staff grade doctor who thought he should see a pain specialist. Following an MRI scan he was told that he had a disc protrusion and may need surgery. He then saw the spine specialist who said there was no indication for surgery and he should learn to live with the situation. Dissatisfied, he requested a further opinion, and his general practitioner referred him to a rheumatologist. He had more physiotherapy which made him worse. He records that he saw nine different hospital doctors about his back pain over a period of 3 years, and they all seemed to give him a different opinion about diagnosis and management. He finally saw a surgeon privately who performed a discectomy. He was no better, but was sure that if the first doctor had made the correct diagnosis of disc protrusion, an earlier operation would have cured him.
>
> This was successfully defended, but when reviewing the problem during a departmental audit, it was obvious that he had been seen by too many different doctors. If he had seen a consultant at his first attendance, and

if a management plan had been developed and explained to him, this litigation might have been avoided. A unit policy was agreed that, because the first visit is the most important for making management decisions, in future patients would generally see a consultant at their first hospital visit.

THE HARMFUL SURGEON

The excessive demands placed on surgeons is now a worrying feature. Long working hours, with a continuous stream of urgent problems, can produce dangerous fatigue and the surgeon is at risk of making mistakes. A good surgeon does not suddenly become harmful overnight. Rather, it is a process. Audit may occasionally identify a 'harmful surgeon', but this is a situation which can be avoided if the surgeon at risk is previously identified.

Self-knowledge

Surgeons are expected to tell senior colleagues about any physical or mental problem which they recognize in themselves and which might reduce their standard of care. When they know that fatigue or stress is reducing their clinical and operative skills, they are expected to devolve clinical responsibility to a similarly qualified colleague. However, most of us are blind to our own faults, and even if we suspect that we can not maintain high standards, confessing it can be humiliating. Some doctors may be reluctant to change life-styles and habits, in spite of the potential risks to patients.

The three most common illnesses which cause a doctor to perform poorly are alcoholism, drug abuse and clinical depression. They are characterized by an insidious onset and lack of insight into one's own condition.

Recognizing harmful colleagues

Doctors are reluctant to 'blow the whistle' on their colleagues, even if they suspect that they are performing badly because they are ill. The problem lies in identifying the sick doctor early enough, and being confident that there is really something wrong. The ill and poorly performing surgeon is difficult to recognize. A Scottish working group described three levels to help doctors identify in themselves or in their colleagues health-related problems [13].

- *Level one*: the worry stage – the doctor may demonstrate worrying behaviour such as poor time-keeping, errors of judgement or unusual irritability. They should be asked to acknowledge a possible problem and seek help.
- *Level two*: the time for action – impaired function, evidence of intense self-criticism, alcohol detected on the breath in the morning. There should be a mandatory discussion within 24 hours, which may result in referral to the medical director.

- *Level three*: the time for immediate action – violence, sensory or motor failing such as impaired hearing or vision. The facts should be determined and the medical director informed at once.

Many doctors are unsure how and when to help a sick colleague, and often resort to the 'old boy' basis which is usually inadequate. One's duty is both to the patient and to the sick or fatigued surgeon. It transcends professional loyalty and the specialist team-spirit. A senior doctor should be informed and the 'sick doctor' policy of the hospital invoked. A number of agencies can help a sick doctor and they are listed at the end of this chapter.

Local factors which are considered to be stress factors for doctors include sleep deprivation, noisy on-call rooms, inadequate provision for meals, poor career counselling and lack of control over one's work. National problems are nursing shortages, pressure of beds and the new business ethos in the National Health Service. These can be responsible for stress, anxiety and burnout.

THE HARMFUL ENVIRONMENT

Surgeons can only provide optimal care when their institutions provide facilities to match the needs of their speciality. Poor surgical results may not be related to the surgeon, but to the environment. And it is the surgeon who is uniquely qualified to judge whether the environment offers the standards for safe patient care. There are several areas of concern, which include

- heavy workload
- informed consent
- time to talk to patients
- communication skills.

Heavy workload

An unacceptably high clinical workload may produce a dangerous environment for the patient. The end result is usually a failure of doctor–patient communications. A relatively innocent and perhaps unavoidable complication can then turn into an unpleasant confrontation and allegations of negligence. When time is at a premium, shared decision making tends to suffer. Patients say that they were not told about the risks, or if they were told they did not understand.

Time for informed consent

Discussion about the merits of surgery is the responsibility of the senior surgeon. It may take several visit to the clinic before the patient is really aware of the value and risks of surgery. Examinations, investigations, discussions and record keeping takes time, but this is quality patient care. Then it is the junior doctor who finally makes sure that the patient has understood the implications of surgery and ensures that a consent form is signed. In a survey of junior doctors who obtained consent for operation, 68%

felt that they had insufficient time to obtain informed consent from patients, and 82% denied having any formal training on the subject [14].

Time to talk and listen

Time is a precious commodity, but it is well spent by staff at all levels if they can be unhurried, and if they can listen to the concerns of anxious patients. The surgeon who sits beside the patient's bed and gives them time to talk – the nurse who pauses to ask the patient how they are today – the houseman who leisurely asks about the situation at home – are all making excellent use of time [11]. There are several studies and reviews which clearly show a correlation between effective communication and improved health outcomes [15]. Doctors who have the skills of communication are not only practising high quality patient care, but unwittingly they help to avoid litigation when there is a surgical complication. Management and staff need to be constantly reminded that time spent talking to patients and relatives is an essential component of good clinical care. Clinics should never be so busy, nor ward rounds so cramped, that there is no time to listen to the patient and their relatives. Genuine kindness makes a tremendous difference [16].

Time for education

Even when time is available, we have to ask if it is being put to optimal use. Most of us could improve our communication skills, learning how to develop relationships whilst gathering relevant data [17]. A number of workshops are now available for clinicians and para-medical staff and management should consider these cost effective [18].

Who is responsible for the environment?

Where audit reveals that the standard of a surgeon's care is consistently poor because of an unsatisfactory environment, appropriate remedial steps should be taken to bring the environment up to an acceptable standard. This may be initiated by surgeons or by management. Surgeons are the custodians of patient care and they are responsible for advising the authorities of deficient facilities and services if they reach an unacceptably low standard. If this is so poor that patients are placed at unnecessary risk, then surgeons may need to reduce their outpatient lists, or refuse to carry out elective operative procedures.

The British Orthopaedic Association Advisory booklet on Consultant Services states that "it is the responsibility of surgeons to see that they are allowed adequate time to talk to and examine the patients, to make certain that they can satisfy the doctrine of 'informed consent' with regard to any treatment that may be offered to the patient, to dictate notes together with letters to the doctor who has sought the consultation, and to teach junior staff or medical students where appropriate" [19]. It is recommended that new patients be allocated 15–20 minutes consultation time, with 30 minutes for each patient seen in tertiary referral clinics.

Undergraduate/graduate education

Doctors who have responsibilities for undergraduate education try to encourage a new generation of doctors to have a spirit of candour, humility and partnership with their patients. These inherent qualities are a now a necessary requirement for entrants into the medical schools, irrespective of a good academic record. They are further developed as an integral part of undergraduate training.

The General Medical Council has recommended that medical ethics and law become a core component of undergraduate education. They advise that the interface between medicine and the law be integrated through the entire curriculum, including the house-officer year [20]. This can also be taught in special study modules lasting a few weeks. In addition, it is an appropriate subject for an intercalated B.Sc. degree, with sufficient topics ranging from legal and ethical aspects of the new genetics, to clinical risk management, medical witness skills and forensic pathology. Universities might offer double degree courses in law and medicine for potential expert witnesses, solicitors, barristers and judges [21].

THE INEXPERIENCED SURGEON

Unexpected operative findings

Sometimes errors occur because the surgeon is not sufficiently experienced for the operation being carried out. In fact, every surgeon will occasionally encounter operative problems which they have not met before. It may be an unexpected pathology, like an unusual tumour, or a complication like massive haemorrhage. It is usually possible to proceed by applying principles learnt in training and recover the situation.

If there is no help readily available and the risks are high then there is a dilemma. Is it in the patient's best interest for the surgeon to continue the operation in this unfamiliar situation, or is it sensible to carry out only essential surgery, close the wound and seek a second opinion with further surgery at a later time? It is a better choice to lose face and admit that the new situation is too difficult, than to subject the patient to unacceptable risk.

Not enough training

Surgeons can often anticipate that an operation might be too difficult for them. It is then good practice to discuss the procedure with a more experienced colleague who may offer to assist the surgeon or at least be available should things go wrong. The alternative is to refer the patient directly to the more experienced doctor, and then assist him in order to learn a new technique. A survey of UK surgeons with an interest in spinal disorders showed that 24% did not regularly carry out spinal decompression; 60% did not carry out posterior fusions and 77% did not do anterior fusions. Spinal deformity was not treated by 90%. However, in spite of their limitations, many expressed an interest in learning new procedures [22]. It is not surprising, therefore, from this data, that unless the choice of surgery is highly selective, some spinal procedures will be carried out by inexperienced surgeons with inevitable complications. Risk management means providing study leave to support the surgeons who wish to learn new procedures.

Part of the responsibility of training junior doctors is to make sure that they are closely supervised. The young doctor's enthusiasm for experience must not run ahead of their surgical skill. There needs to be particular vigilance with a new trainee, when the consultant is on holiday or when locum surgeons are employed.

Case Report 35: Not enough experience. Mr JJ was a 44-year-old achondroplastic with spinal stenosis. He had had low back pain for 15 years but, in the past 12 months, walking had become difficult because his legs would go numb after walking about 200 m. He was referred to a spinal surgeon who correctly made the diagnosis of spinal stenosis and neurogenic claudication. He carried out an MRI scan which showed stenosis throughout the lower thoracic and lumbar spine. It was most marked at L2/3/4 levels.

Mr JJ remembers being told that without surgery he would probably go off his feet and, although the operation was not without risk, he could expect to be able to walk comfortably again and be relieved of some of his back pain. He does not remember being told of any serious risk.

During the operation the surgeon used spinal cord monitoring and, when starting to operate at L2 level, there were signs of loss of signal. The operation was discontinued. Mr JJ awoke from the operation to find his legs paralysed and he had lost control of his bladder and bowels.

He claimed that the surgeon had treated him negligently by failing to warn him of a serious neurological risk, and failing to refer him to a specialist centre where others had more experience on operating on achondroplastics with stenosis.

There was debate about whether Mr JJ had been told about the risk of paraplegia. The surgeon conceded that this was his first patient with achondroplasia. However, it was agreed that in any event, even in expert hands, the same complication would probably have occurred, and even without surgery his condition would have been much the same within 2 years. A small settlement was made out of court.

REFERENCES

1. Vincent CA, Pincus T, Scurr JH, *et al.* Patient's experience of surgical accidents *Qual. Health Care* 1993; 2: 77–82.
2. Charles SC, Wilbert JR, Franke KJ. Sued and non-sued physicians self reported reactions to malpractice litigation *Am. J. Psychiat.* 1985; 192: 437.

3. Ennis M Grudzinskas JG. The effects of accidents and litigation on doctors In: Vincent CA Ennis M Audley RJ ed. *Medical Accidents* Oxford. Oxford University Press, 1993.

4. Firth-Cozens J Stress, psychological problems and clinical performance. In: Vincent CA, Ennis M and Audley RJ Eds *Medical Accidents* Oxford: Oxford University Press 1993.

5. NHS Executive *Clinical Negligence Costs* London: Department of Health 1996; FDL (96) 39.

6. Heasell S. Victims do not always take precedence *BMJ* 1998; 316: 73–74.

7. Cowell HR. Wrong-site surgery *J. Bone. Jt. Surg.* 1998; 80-A: 463.

8. Foubister G, Hughes SPF. Fractures of the femoral neck: a retrospective and prospective study *J. R. Coll. Surg. Edinburgh* 1989; 34: 249–252.

9. Wenger NS, Lieberman JR. An assessment of orthopaedic surgeons' knowledge of medical ethics. *J. Bone. Jt. Surg.* 1998; 80-A, 198–206.

10. *Checklist for Anaesthetic Apparatus* published by The Association of Anaesthetists of Great Britain and Ireland, 9, Bedford Square, London WC1B 3RA, 1997.

11. Rosen A. Last on the list. Personal view *BMJ* 1998; 316: 1324–1325

12. Johnson JN. Making self-regulation credible *BMJ* 1998; 316: 1847–1848.

13. Beecham L. Doctors with health problems should seek help *BMJ* 1998; 316: 1412.

14. Richardson N, Jones P, Thomas M. Should house officers obtain consent for operations and anaesthesia? *Health Trends* 1996; 28: 56–59.

15. Meryn S. Improving doctor–patient communication *BMJ* 1998; 316: 1922.

16. Short D. Show God's kindness today *Triple Helix*, published by Christian Medical Fellowship Spring 1998; 3.

17. Bird J, Cohnen-Cole SA. The three function model of the medical interview *Adv. Psychosom. Med.* 1990; 20: 65–88.

18. Bird J, Hall A, Maguirte P, *et al.* Workshops for consultants on teaching of clinical communication skills *Med. Educ.* 1993; 27: 181–185.

19. *Advisory Booklet on Consultant Orthopaedic and Trauma Services* British Orthopaedic Association 1990; 20.

20. Doyal L, Gillon R. Medical ethics and law as a core subject in medical education *BMJ* 1998; 316: 1623–1624.

21. Richards P, Kennedy IM, Lord Woolf. Managing medical mishaps *BMJ* 1996; 313: 243–244.

22. Okafor BE, Sullivan MF. Survey of spinal theraputic procedures in the United Kingdom *Eur. Spine* 1997; 6: 294–297.

AGENCIES TO HELP A SICK DOCTOR

- The Sick Doctor's Trust (Tel. 0123 234 5163) for addictive physicians.
- The British Doctor's and Dentist's Group (Tel. 0171 487 4445) for drug and alcohol misuse.
- Overseas Doctors Association (Tel. 0161 236 5594).
- BMA 24 Hour Stress Counselling Service (Tel. 0645 200169).
- National Counselling Service for Sick Doctors (Tel. 0171 935 5982).
- Doctor's Support Network (Tel. 0171 727 3738) self-help group/mental health problems.

GLOSSARY

ANNULUS: the tough outer part of the intervertebral disc. It is a layered structure, like onion skin. Axial loading of the spine causes the annulus to bulge outwards, whilst it supports the inner nucleus of the disc. This arrangement makes a healthy disc stronger to axial load than the bone of the vertebrae.

APOPHYSEAL JOINT: synonymous with facet joint.

ARACHNOID: the thin delicate membrane which lines the inside of the dural membrane in the vertebral canal. The spinal cord above L2 and the cauda equina below L2 lie within the arachnoid and dural sac, and are bathed in cerebro-spinal fluid.

ARACHNOIDITIS: painful inflammation of the arachnoid, which causes fibrous scarring of the cauda equina.

AXONS: the small nerve fibres. A bundle of axons form the nerve trunk.

CAUDA EQUINA: the several nerve roots in the lower part of the spinal canal below L2. The sacral roots are positioned towards the mid-line posteriorly, and are at risk if the dura is damaged in the mid-line.

CEREBRO-SPINAL FLUID: the clear fluid secreted in the brain, which surrounds the spinal cord and the cauda equina within the arachnoid and dura.

CHYMOPAPAIN: a lysing agent that can be injected into the nucleus of the intervertebral disc to shrink the size of the disc. It is appropriate therapy if the disc is not sequestrated. It has the occasional complication of anaphylactic shock, but results are comparable with open disc surgery.

COCCYX: the tail-bone of the spine below the sacrum, made up of several segments. If traumatized it is responsible for unpleasant pain, but this usually resolves. Persistent coccygeal pain (coccydinia) is considered to be inappropriate.

COMPUTERIZED TOMOGRAPHY (CT): an imaging modality using computerized X-rays. It is particularly good at imaging bone, and will demonstrate disc protrusion with about 95% accuracy.

CONGENITAL: present at birth.

CROSS-LEG PAIN: a modification of the straight leg raising test. It is positive if, when the painless leg is lifted off the couch, pain is felt in the symptomatic leg. It is a classical sign of prolapsed intervertebral disc.

DEGENERATION: wear-and-tear changes in bone or soft tissues.

DEGENERATIVE SPONDYLOLISTHESIS: a forward displacement of one vertebra on another in association with degenerative changes. In contrast to isthmic spondylolisthesis, the neural arch is intact. It is most common at L4/5 level and is more common in women than in men. It develops in the fifth decade of life and generally causes back pain. If there is some spinal stenosis, the dural sac and its contents are compressed. If one nerve root is irritated it will cause sciatica with root entrapment pain. If there is also stenosis at another level, multiple level stenosis can cause neurogenic claudication.

DORSAL NERVE ROOT: that component of the nerve root which contains the sensory fibres from the limb to the spinal cord. It is on the dorsal (posterior) aspect of the nerve root.

DURA: the tough membrane on the outside of the arachnoid extending from the top to the bottom of the spine. It is sometimes torn during spinal surgery, and if the arachnoid is also torn, there is a leakage of cerebro-spinal fluid.

DURAL SLEEVE: an extension of the dural sac covering the proximal part of the nerve roots. It is compressed and its image obliterated in a radiculogram if a disc protrusion presses on the root.

EXTRUSION: part of the fragment of a disc protrusion is extruded outside the annulus, whilst part remains within the disc space.

FACET JOINTS: the small joints at the back of the vertebrae which link the segments together. Sometimes called apophyseal joints. The spine is a three-joint system and, if there is disc degeneration, the facet joints also tend to be degenerate. These changes are common and are often asymptomatic.

FEMORAL STRETCH TEST: this is recorded as the patient lies face down. The knee is bent and the thigh lifted backwards off the couch. It is a root tension sign and, if painful, suggests a disc protrusion affecting the L3 or L4 nerve root. Only 5% of disc protrusion are at this level (L3/4) with this sign, whilst 95% are at L4/5 or L5/S1.

FENESTRATION: the surgical removal of a small piece of bone in the lamina making a 'window' to gain access to the vertebral canal.

FISTULA: a false passage between two structures. For example, between the dural sac and the surface of the skin (cerebro-spinal fluid fistula) or between an artery and vein (arterio-venous fistula), the bladder and the bowel (recto-vesical fistula).

GANGLION: a swelling of nerve tissue on the dorsal root within the spinal canal which contains nerve cells.

HOLMAN'S SIGN: a clinical sign of deep venous thrombosis. When the foot is passively dorsiflexed – pulled upwards – the patient feels pain in the calf.

ILIAC CREST: the iliac bone is a component of the pelvis – the large plate of bone which is attached to the sacrum by the sacroiliac joint. The iliac crest is the superior (upper) part of the iliac bone. It is a useful source of donor bone for a bone graft.

INTERMITTENT CLAUDICATION: a clinical condition when a patient has pain in the legs when walking which is relieved by rest. It is caused by peripheral vascular disease in the arteries of the legs.

INTERVERTEBRAL FORAMEN: the outer boundary of the root canal, composed of the vertebra above, the vertebra below and the disc in front. The nerve root passes through the foramen into the soft tissues.

ISTHMIC SPONDYLOLISTHESIS: a condition where one vertebra is displaced forwards on the lower vertebra. There is a defect in the neural arch, allowing the body of the vertebra to displace forwards, whilst the lamina of the neural arch remains behind. The canal is therefore widened. It occurs in 5% of the population and is often symptomless. A mechanical strain can weaken the fibrous tissue supporting the bony defect and the patient may then experience back pain. If chronic it can be helped by a spinal fusion. Sometimes bony thickening at the site of the defect will irritate a nerve root causing sciatica – 'root entrapment syndrome'.

KYPHOSIS: an arching of the spine forwards. The thoracic spine has a normal kyphosis. This can be exaggerated in osteoporotic women if there are multiple compression fractures.

LAMINA: the plate of bone at the back of the vertebra arching over the spinal canal. A lamina on each side unites in the mid-line at the spinous process.

LAMINECTOMY: a surgical term to describe removal of a whole lamina. The neural arch is then incomplete. Is sometimes used incorrectly to describe a fenestration.

LATERAL RECESS: the lateral part of the central canal at the level of the pedicle. An oval-shaped spinal canal does not have a lateral recess. A trefoil canal has a lateral recess in its lateral part. The nerve root leaving the canal at the next lower inter-space is situated in the lateral recess. Entrapment of the nerve root at this site can cause 'root entrapment syndrome'.

LIGAMENTUM FLAVUM: the strong ligament linking each vertebra to the next, from lamina to lamina, at the back of the spinal canal. It is a yellow ligament that has to be cut open to expose the dural sac, the nerve roots and a protruding disc.

LIST: when the spine is twisted to one side, usually as a result of disc protrusion. It is induced by gravity and is abolished by lying down.

LORDOSIS: an arching backwards of the spine. The lumbar and cervical spines are normally lordotic.

MAGNETIC RESONANCE IMAGING (MRI): uses magnetism and radio-waves to image the body. It is particularly good at imaging soft tissues, and is the imaging modality of choice for the spine. It has a 97% accuracy for imaging disc protrusion.

MYELOGRAM: a spinal X-ray where radio-opaque dye is injected into the dural sac. It outlines the dural sac, and can identify a bulging disc with about 90% accuracy for L3/4 and L4/5 levels. It has about 70% accuracy for L5/S1.

NERVE ROOT: the combined anterior and posterior root in the spinal canal. A nerve root leaves the canal at each level. The bundle of nerve roots below L2 is called the cauda equina.

NEURAL ARCH: the posterior part of the spinal canal composed of the pedicles on each side laterally, and the laminae posteriorly.

NEUROGENIC CLAUDICATION: a clinical condition where the patient has pain or discomfort in one or both legs when they walk, as a result of spinal stenosis. Pain begins after a short distance until the patient has to stop. The discomfort is then relieved and they can walk again. It is unusual under 50 years of age. There is usually more than one level of stenosis. The nerve roots between two levels of stenosis become congested with venous blood and, when a patient wants to walk, this probably causes a failure of arterial vasodilatation and impaired nerve function. If symptoms are severe it can often be relieved by spinal decompression, although a trial of calcitonin is worth considering prior to offering surgery.

NUCLEUS PULPOSUS: the central part of the intervertebral disc, within the peripheral annulus.

ODONTOID: the odontoid process is the bony projection from C2 vertebra (the axis) which extends vertically into C1 (the atlas). It is held in place by the strong transverse ligament of the atlas. It lies anterior to the spinal cord. Fractures of the odontoid are classified into three types according to their position.

OSTEOPHYTE: a pathological prominence of bone which develops in association with degenerative change. Osteophytes are a sign of 'wear and tear'. They tend to grow into the ligamentous attachments at the edge of the vertebral bodies. They are very common in the asymptomatic elderly population.

OSTEOPOROSIS: loss of bone mass. The quality of the bone is normal, but there is not enough of it. Osteoporosis increases with age, with 1% bone loss each year after 45 years of age. Those most affected are at risk of fracture in old age.

PARASTHESIA: pins and needles or a sensation of numbness.

PARS INTERARTICULARIS: a fibrous defect in the neural arch where there is a loss of bony continuity. It is present in about 5% of the population, and is often symptomless. It is the cause of isthmic spondylolisthesis.

PEDICLES: the bony struts which project backwards from the vertebral bodies to join the laminae. They form the lateral part of the vertebral canal.

POSTERIOR LONGITUDINAL LIGAMENT: the long ligament which links the vertebral bodies together behind each vertebra. This ligament is the immediate posterior boundary of the vertebral canal. A bulging disc stretches this ligament. A ruptured disc may extrude through the ligament, or pass between the ligament and bone to be 'sub-ligamentous'.

PROGNOSIS: the probable outcome of a condition.

PROTRUSION: a term applied to a bulging disc when the peripheral annulus is intact, but is bulging backwards into the vertebral canal. A disc protrusion occurs after there has been a long-standing degenerative process. The nucleus of the disc becomes fissured. Multiple fissures result in fragmentation of the nucleus and, when a fragment has formed, the disc is prone to protrude under a fairly minimal load. The fragment is squeezed backwards tearing the inner annulus and this causes the disc to bulge.

PSEUDOMENINGOCELE: a false posterior extension of the dural sac which can occur post-operatively if the dura has been torn. MR imaging shows that it is quite common in a mild form and it is usually asymptomatic. It is a cause of post-operative pain or bladder symptoms if nerve roots are intermittently trapped in the neck of the sac.

RADICULOGRAM: synonymous with myelogram. It visualizes the nerve roots.

ROOT CANAL: that part of the vertebral canal which contains the nerve root from its leaving the main component of the dural sac. It extends from the inner side of the pedicle to the intervertebral foramen.

ROOT ENTRAPMENT SYNDROME: a clinical condition causing severe root pain in the leg usually down to the ankle and foot – sciatica. The pain is in the same distribution as the pain of disc protrusion, but the cause is different. There is bony or soft tissue degenerative change in the root canal compromising the nerve root. The pain usually starts insidiously, and becomes quite severe and constant. It can slowly resolve with time but, if bad enough, surgical decompression is indicated.

SACRAL ROOTS: there are four pairs of sacral roots which continue into the sacral vertebral canal from the lumbar region. These supply the bladder and bowel and sexual function, the skin around the anus and the anal sphincter.

SACRUM: the bony part of the spine distal to the lumbar spine and above the coccyx. It is segmental in nature.

SCOLIOSIS: a twisted spine which, when observed from behind, looks like a letter 'S'.

SEQUESTRATION: a term used to describe a fragment of disc which has passed through the torn annulus, and is lying either free within the vertebral canal or in a sub-ligamentous position.

SPASM: a term applied to muscles when they contract involuntarily. The spasm is visible and palpable. It occurs in the presence of infection and tumour. It causes a list in disc protrusion. It may be imitated by voluntary contraction.

SPINA BIFIDA: a condition where the neural arch is incomplete. The spinous process is usually absent or bifid, and the resulting gap in the neural arch is replaced by fibrous tissue. It occurs in about 10% of the population and is thought to be clinically insignificant. Spina bifida occulta occurs when the skin is intact. Spina bifida overta occurs when there is loss of skin and soft tissue over the bony defect exposing the nerve roots. This is a serious condition usually associated with some paralysis, requiring surgery at birth.

SPINAL CANAL: synonymous with vertebral canal.

SPINAL STENOSIS: an anatomical term used to describe a small spinal canal. When a small canal is compromised by a disc protrusion or by degenerative change, it can be responsible for symptoms.

SPINOUS PROCESS: the bony projection from the back of the vertebral laminae to which muscles and ligaments are attached.

SPONDYLOLISTHESIS: a forward displacement of one vertebra on another. Isthmic spondylolisthesis tends to occur at L5/S1 and is a result of pars defects in the neural arch. Degenerative spondylolisthesis is more common at L4/5 and is a forward displacement with an intact neural arch. Traumatic spondylolisthesis follows fracture of the neural arch.

SPONDYLOLYSIS: a condition where there are pars defects in the neural arch, but no forward displacement of the vertebra.

STRAIGHT LEG RAISING (SLR): a test lifting the straight leg as the patient lies flat on the couch. It is a root tension sign and, when limited, suggests disc protrusion.

SYNDROME: a collection of symptoms which together define a condition, i.e. 'root entrapment syndrome'.

TRANSVERSE PROCESS: the bony projection from the side of the vertebra to which muscles and ligaments are attached.

VENTRAL NERVE ROOT: that component of the nerve root which supplies the motor fibres from the spinal cord to the limb. It is on the ventral (anterior) aspect of the nerve root.

VERTEBRAL BODY: the large block of bone anterior to the vertebral canal, attached to the next vertebral body by the intervertebral disc.

VERTEBRAL CANAL: synonymous with the spinal canal, it is the tunnel behind the vertebral bodies and the discs, which contains the spinal cord above L2 and the cauda equina below L2.

INDEX